ILLNESS AND HEALING

IN THE CONTEXT OF COSMIC EVOLUTION

DR RITA LEROI

Illness and Healing
in the context
of Cosmic Evolution

Translated by
Anna Meuss

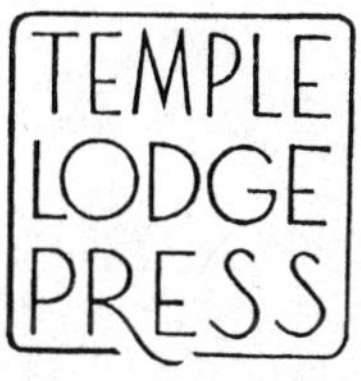

First English Edition 1988

© R. Leroi and A. Meuss 1988

Cover design by Paulo Frank Boer

British Library Cataloguing
in Publication Data:

LEROI, Rita
Illness and Healing
1. Man. Sickness. Spiritual Aspects
I. Title
291.4

ISBN 0-904693-15-5

Typeset by Temple Lodge Press London
Printed in Great Britain by
Whitstable Litho Kent

CONTENTS

TRANSLATOR'S PREFACE

Until her death in September 1988 at the age of 74, Dr Rita Leroi regularly took up the impulse given by Dr Ita Wegman, the first leader of the Medical Section at the Goetheanum, to take the medical work of Rudolf Steiner to all parts of the world. Every year she set out to visit a number of ccuntries in different continents. In the last year of her life, for example, she visited Namibia, South Africa, Australia and New Zealand, and gave about 70 lectures on 20 different medical subjects during the tour. Some months before she set out on each of her tours I was usually asked to translate the lectures she intended to give in English. These were addressed to four different groups of people – members of the medical profession who are interested in the anthroposophical approach to medicine, anthroposophical doctors, members of the Anthroposophical Society, and interested non-members. Dr Leroi, who by the way had a very good command of the English language, then studied the translations thoroughly and made them her own before she began her journey.

I count it a privilege to have been asked to translate these lectures, for each of them reflects years of effort in penetrating the works of Rudolf Steiner and relating them in a living way to the real needs of patients. The lectures to the medical profession also reveal considerable experience in communicating anthroposophical medicine to the medical profession without compromising it. At the same time each lecture is carefully thought out to meet the needs of the particular group of people who are being addressed and, last but not least, each has the air of a work of art, giving the translator – and it is hoped also the reader – a feeling of satisfaction on perceiving the rounded balance of the whole. It is therefore a great pleasure to know that this small volume will make five of Dr Leroi's lectures available to a wider English-language readership.

Their sources are as follows: 'Illness and the Overcoming of Evil' was originally given as a lecture entitled, *'Der Krankheitsprozess und das Böse' (Kunstseminar*, Vienna, November 1986). 'Overcoming the Ahrimanic Element in the Human Organism' was originally given as *'Der Aetherleib zwischen Kosmos und Erde'* (*Krebstagung* 1981) and published in *Beiträge zu einer Erweiterung der Heilkunst nach geisteswissenschaftlichen Erkenntnissen*, *Heft* 2, 1987. 'Sacrifice and Healing' was originally given as *'Das Wirken von Merkur-Raphael'* (*Krebstagung*, 16 September 1982) and published in *Beiträge*, *Heft* 2, 1987. 'The Power of the Human Ego: from Darkness to Light' was orginally given as *'Lichtprozesse im Menschen'* (*Krebstagung*, 19 September 1985). 'Gifts of Earth and Cosmos: the Healing Power of Antimony' was originally given as *'Antimon'* in Bad Liebenzell, April 1982, published in *Beiträge*, *Heft* 6, 1983.

Anna Meuss

Illness and Healing

in the context

of Cosmic Evolution

CHAPTER 1

ILLNESS AND THE OVERCOMING OF EVIL

It is surprising to find, on reflection, that the idea of malignancy, of evil, occurs only with reference to cancer in medicine. Medical terms often sound quite dramatic, for instance: pernicious (liable to be fatal) anaemia, galloping consumption, circulatory collapse, dumping syndrome, stroke or cerebrovascular accident (the Swiss speak of this as being preceded by a *Berührung*, a touch, and this suggests awareness of the angel who comes to give warning of death, lightly touching the person concerned.'

The term 'malignant' on the other hand is generally reserved for tumours showing invasive and destructive growth, egotistically having things their own way, breaking organic boundaries regardless and destroying the human form. All kinds of moral concepts come up in connection with this disease. Sigmund, a brilliant pathologist, consciously or unconsciously hit the nail on the head when he called cancer a 'catastrophe of form'.

To get any further with this, we must first of all bring to mind the different principles which constitute the human being. The physical body is the most perfect of these. The most sublime spirits have been working on it through the aeons, sacrificing themselves to complete this marvellous building, the temple of the godhead. Even today they devote themselves to its continued maintenance, building it up again and restoring it while we are asleep. Every morning when we wake up we can experience the miracle they have achieved, feeling quickened and refreshed. The living physical body is constantly being healed, indeed we may say hallowed, by those cosmic spirits.

The etheric body is of more recent origin. It was the gift of the Sun stage of evolution. It warms, it glows in all colours, sounding in the music of the spheres and bringing life. It is intimately bound up in its functions with the physical body and it may be said to provide the medium for the constructive work done by the cosmic hierarchies during the night. This is a vital necessity, for the astral body with its emotions, desires and passions is constantly attacking the marvellous building which is our organism. The astral body is still far from fully developed, and any kind of activity in our souls – thinking, intense feelings, will impulses – causes destruction. Only the heart, our central organ which is also the centre point of all etheric streams, can equalize, compensate for, those attacks which continue for decades. Night after night, the constructive forces of the cosmic world also stream into the heart.

We may ask ourselves whether there is any point to such constant constructive and destructive activity. Well, the point is that we must be given opportunity to fulfil our karma and develop the youngest of the constituent principles in the human being, which is the ego. This has potential to achieve the highest and it ranks above all the others. The ego needs to be exposed to the vicissitudes of life if it is to gain strength. The contribution we make to world evolution will be all the greater the more we transform this constituent element of the human being and do so in full awareness, making it come closer to its archetype and paradigm.

Now there is one issue that simply has to be faced. It is the question of the nature of evil. It is not my intention to go into long philosophical discussions on the subject. Basing ourselves on Rudolf Steiner, the answer may be summed up as follows: Anything acting at the wrong time and in the wrong place or wrong sphere has evil consequences. Thus there is Lucifer, who always wants to hold on to the past – in obsolete social forms such as dictatorships, for instance – rather than work towards true community. And there is Ahriman, who comes up with premature inventions at a time when humanity is not yet ready for them, atomic power being an example.

The human mind desires to acquire as much knowledge as possible and that is a good thing; if however this desire shifts to the sphere of the will and concentrates on material things we call it thieving. I know the philosophers among you will consider this an oversimplified definition of evil, but it is a useful one. Every good thing becomes a bad thing if taken to excess. Considering human virtues, therefore: generosity becomes profligacy, economy avarice, courage rashness, patience inertia, and tolerance turns to uncritical acceptance. How does the change from good to evil come about?

The German writer and playwright Lessing demonstrated this very well in his *Faust* fragment. Faust demanded the services of the fleetest of the infernal spirits. Seven spirits appeared in response to his incantation. 'Which of you is the swiftest?' he asked. All seven shouted, 'I am!' (Surprisingly, only six of the seven devils were liars.) Then each stepped forward to boast how swift he could be, viz:

    as the wind
    as light
    as a thought
    as the arrow of the plague
    as the avenger's hand

'Not one of them is swift enough,' Faust said. Then the last of the seven stepped forward: 'I am as swift as the change from good to evil.' 'You are the devil for me, for nothing is swifter than that. I know this from experience.' A profound truth. It also shows very clearly that the secret of evil has to do with the question of balance. Goodness is a highly unstable middle state. At any moment it may go to the luciferic or the ahrimanic extreme. Just think how quickly loving devotion turns into the crassest egotism, how quickly the search for knowledge becomes vainglory, and a positive initiative turns to ambition. Only we ourselves know how quickly this happens. Others do not notice it until later. If we catch the moment, it will be possible to turn back. Lessing's Faust had not grasped this.

What does it all mean? It means that the ego, and only the ego, is the weight that tips the scales, that it alone can make the balance go one way or the other. This core of our being, grown wholly independent of the divine guidance, constantly has to struggle to maintain the balance. Human beings had to be given such an unstable lower ego that is capable of error and over and over again swings from good to evil and back again, so that they will be able to attain to the higher ego by their very own efforts. That is the only way in which human beings can also have 'free will'.

This takes us back to the evil in cancer. Modern scientists are still one-sidedly fixing their attention on the cell. Let us first of all hear what Rudolf Steiner has to say:

What is a cell? A cell is something with a mind of its own that stands out against what the human being represents. It has its own way of growing, its own life. If you consider on the one hand the whole form of the human being as it has been fashioned by powers prevailing on earth and powers from beyond this earth, and then somehow come to consider the cell, it is the cell which upsets the applecart for those primary powers. It actually destroys those external powers, wanting to develop a life of its own. Even under normal conditions we are constantly waging war in our organisms against the life of the cell. The absurdest of views has arisen in connection with therapy and physiology at cellular level, with the cell consistently regarded as the primary element and the human organism as a construct of cells. In reality the human being is a whole and as such connected with the cosmos, and is for ever involved in the struggle against the self-will of the cell. It is actually the cell which is constantly causing disruption in the organism; it does not play a constructive role.

So here we have the original polarity of form and substance, of organism and cell. What is the true nature of the cell? How should we regard the organism in this context?

Each of the three higher principles of the human being, the etheric body, the astral body and the ego has a role to play in physical development and also in the sphere of soul and spirit. They form a hierarchic order. The etheric body may be said to draw the basic design of the individual person we are at this time, the astral body to fill in the detail inwardly by developing the organs, and the ego to give the final touches to the outer form of this work of art which is our body, using the blood as its instrument to maintain the equilibrium of internal functions. Every single cell bears the stamp of the ego organization, down to its smallest detail.

In the sphere of soul and spirit, the etheric body comes to expression in our ability to think, the astral body in feeling, and the ego in will activity. We are consciously aware of these faculties and able to control them. The physical functions of those higher principles are however largely at an unconscious level. They are guided and inspired by cosmic powers, the spirits of the hierarchies. Rudolf Steiner referred to these powers when speaking of the organism as a system of forces that constantly brings the human form, a purely spiritual principle, to realization, using cell substance as its material.

And yet what is a cell? In far distant times, during the polar epoch of the earth, the human body consisted entirely of life ether. This body evolved further, but certain individuals did not enter into further evolution. They remained behind and grew stunted. Later, single-celled animals developed from them and also the cells on which more complex life forms are based. The life ether provides for the faculty of procreation, that is, of reproducing ourselves in like form. That is the specific faculty a cell has, and it is the only one. Anything which has to do with a cell assuming a particular form and differentiated functions derives from the powers which govern the organism, as defined above. It is essentially incorrect to say that organisms are made up of cells. They differentiate into cells. Let me quote two modern scientists. First of all the anatomist Blechschmidt:

> Again and again the question is put as to why a human ovum develops into a human being. But this is based on the wrong premise. A human being does not become a human being, but *is* a human being, at every stage of development in fact. Humanness is therefore something that goes beyond the sphere of matter, yet constantly intervenes in the organism as this grows and comes into being, to provide guidance and establish order.

The zoologist Adolf Portmann said:

> Biologists are getting to be at home in the sphere of the invisible. Here no organism is ever built up from cells. A plasmatic coherent whole, persisting as such through all stages of development, differentiates itself . . . The study of microscopic structures and of forms arising at a level that is not visible is today taking us to the actual site where form is created. We do have some idea that we are speaking of a great mystery when we say glibly: 'An organism builds itself from an

ovum.' Who is it that thus builds itself? We come upon the riddle of the 'self' – one that we are bound to come up against over and over again.

Why is it that all our life we have to struggle against the life of the cell? Because cells are entities that have remained behind and the proliferative life ether forces of the Ancient Moon are active in them. Forces of a past period are projecting into normal evolution, providing the material for the creative powers. If those creative powers weaken, if the ego, astral body and etheric body are not sufficiently active, the cell element slips from the grasp of those higher principles, gains the upper hand and proliferates. In the process it destroys the marvellous form of the physical body, and this is why we call cancer evil or malignant. The balance between spirit and matter has been profoundly upset, with matter gaining the ascendancy.

The essential principle behind all matter is Ahriman. He remained behind in the Earth region when the Moon separated from the earth. He and his helpers reside beneath the solid surface of the earth and at the present time make every effort, night after night, to let the earth ether, the life ether of the past age which is full of proliferative tendencies, penetrate the physical and etheric bodies of human beings as they lie asleep. If they were to succeed entirely, immortal, for ever earth-bound spectres of human beings would result which are no longer open to the intervention of the higher principles of human nature. Rudolf Steiner made it clear that this only happened very rarely. But the ahrimanic adversaries do achieve partial victories in parts of the body where the higher principles are not properly incarnated and unable to make their mark. Malignant tumours will arise in those sites as the cell principle emancipates in all its egotism. However, whilst the change from good to evil may occur at the speed of lightning in the sphere of the soul and spirit, it does take more time in the organic sphere. This makes it possible for us to intervene in the process of cancer development, for cancer is a disease that often takes many years, even decades, to develop. We can come in and help at any time to bring about a change of direction.

Acute inflammation is the direct opposite of a malignant tumour. In this case, the balance has shifted in favour of the luciferic principle. Maximum activity is developed by all the constituent principles in the human being: the ego acts through heat, i.e. fever, the astral body through pain, the etheric body in a fortissimo of circulation, and the physical body through swelling. Mediaeval physicians already knew *calor*, *dolor*, *rubor*, and *tumor* (heat, pain, redness and swelling) to be the cardinal symptoms of acute inflammatory conditions. As healing ensues, pus is formed. Pus in itself is a healing process, and this kind of pus used to be called *pus bonum et laudabile*, good and laudable pus.

During all the centuries when Lucifer was the one to lead mankind astray – I am referring to the Graeco-Roman period – highly febrile conditions were the order of the day. Even if they proved fatal they were never considered malignant, for every acute in-flammation has a tendency to heal spon-taneously. In the case of cancer, on the other hand, nothing happens, the constituent principles have grown immobile, have withdrawn, and the individual has subnormal temperatures. The ego, which lives in the sphere of warmth, has grown blind to the enemy. The tumour develops insidiously. a dark, chill disease that never heals of its own accord.

We oppose this process with mistletoe therapy. This activates all the constituent principles. It creates a mildly febrile state in the individual, not only physically but also in soul and spirit. The result is that he or she regains interest in the world around, is able to warm to enthusiasm again, and becomes capable of developing initiative and acting out of this.

If it proves impossible to overcome cancer, despite the fact that every available method has been used, the wisdom that orders the world ordains the following (I am quoting from Rudolf Steiner):

The body collapses, so that it may sweat out, if I may put it like that, the unrightful etheric processes that it has taken into itself under the ahrimanic influence. This will give you an idea of cancer which may be paradoxical but is nevertheless correct. In many cases it is the only means available to the powers of good if they are to save the individual from the clutches of Ahriman.

Let me add that in this case Ahriman is 'part of that power desiring evil that always produces good.'

We can now see more clearly why this disease is the only one to be called 'malignant' and why Rudolf Steiner spoke of the physical powers rebelling against the powers of the human etheric body. Those physical powers become enemies, and there will be some place where the sacred temple of the physical body is made alien to the higher principles and spiritual powers that impose human form. The 'catastrophe of form' consists in adversary powers taking over territory.

What we perceive to be the human form is a manifestation of sublime spiritual powers. Goethe had some intuition of this when he spoke the following words as he contemplated Schiller's skull in the charnel house:

> Yet I, an adept, could read what
>   was writ
> In sacred letters not perceived by all,
> When in the midst of massed rigidity
> A form of untold splendour I beheld.
> There in that narrow room of cold decay,
> A breath of freedom and reviving warmth
> Did come to me as life sprung forth
>   from death.
> Ah, the delight of that mysterious form!
> Divine thought leaving here its trace.
> A sight that yonder ocean brought to
>   mind
> Where flows the very essence of all form.

Goethe penetrated so far as to perceive the creative power of the etheric world. This is 'the ocean where flows the very essence of all form.'

All illnesses arise because the harmony between the constituent principles is disturb- ed. In the case of cancer, however, there is a profound difference. Rudolf Steiner referred to this when he said:

It is incorrect to call tumours neoplasms, new growths. They are new only in the sense that they did not exist before. They are not new in so far as they grow in the soil of the organism itself, which is contained within its skin.

They are in fact not part of the human being, but foreign bodies in the literal sense of the word, aggressive, chaotic growths which have nothing to do with the image of God.

The above essentially provides the basis for the whole approach to treatment and prevention. This disease – relatively un- common in the past but now the disease of our time, because ahrimanic powers are in the ascendancy – challenges the power of our egoity with its malignancy. Demons are making themselves at home on abandoned altars. In regions where the ego forces are not fully effective the astral body de- generates, the etheric body becomes para- lysed, the balance is upset and malignancy develops. If we merely remove the malignant cells of the tumour – which is the method used in conventional medicine – we have not really cured the patient. What have we to offer instead? We are indeed fortunate to have the whole of Rudolf Steiner's work as our therapy, for this encompasses the way to bring up children, education, religious renewal, eurythmy as a new art of movement, a renewal of medicine and the whole of science, biodynamic agriculture and nu- trition, the threefold social order – the whole wide range is available and only waiting for us to take it up and enter into intense practical exercise.

The help we need to strengthen the constituent principles of our human nature can be found in all those different fields. These principles will then become better and better doors through which strength may enter during the night. That is genuine prevention, genuine therapy. Courage then arises to build a strong bastion to protect us from 'evil', not only for ourselves, but for our brothers and sisters in all parts of the world.

Last but not least Rudolf Steiner gave us mistletoe as a causal medicament to strengthen the creative cosmic powers in the organism and subdue foreign substance. We may be able to triumph over the disease in this life or we may not, but we shall always be able to bring healing in some form or other to our patients when we use this therapy. Mistletoe therapy with Iscador helps patients to reach that inner turning point that enables them to move towards a new state of balance as the ego gains in strength. Again and again patients come and tell us: 'I am glad I developed this illness. If destiny had not brought this about, I should never have gained such depth to my life and in my relationships to others.' 'Now I am ready,' a desperately ill woman said to me with a smile. 'There is new meaning to my life,' were the words of a young physician who had just undergone surgery. 'It is a great blessing to experience this illness, the most marvellous thing a physician may know.'

Let us consider the group Rudolf Steiner sculpted in wood, where we see the representative of humanity. It pictures the Mercury period of the earth in which we are today and have been ever since the Mystery of Golgotha. Christ is the true Mercury, the true healer, joining heaven and earth. Stepping forth in freedom, foregoing the exercise of power, He establishes the balance between opposing powers purely through the sunlike greatness of his very nature. He is love incarnate and we recognize in Him the healer of all worlds. If we follow Christ and transform our ego so that it can master our powers of soul, maintaining the balance among them, if we come awake in perceiving the needs of others and seeing that they are different, we are contributing, however humbly, to the future of the human race and of the divine world.

CHAPTER 2

OVERCOMING THE AHRIMANIC ELEMENT IN THE HUMAN ORGANISM

Rudolf Steiner has given many indications that may serve to deepen our understanding of the cancer process, and he provided an accurate description of how cancer develops in relation to the four constituent principles of the human being which he called the physical, etheric and astral bodies and the ego. There are however two statements he made concerning the etheric body that appear to be contradictory. In the first course of lectures that he gave for members of the medical profession he said:

> Tumours arise in a situation where certain processes in the physical body appear to be in direct opposition to the activity of the etheric body; processes in the physical body appear to be rebelling, as it were, against the activity of the etheric body, so that the etheric body is no longer able to take effective action in these areas of the physical body.

In one of the last lectures he gave in London he said:

> We cannot grasp the idea of a carcinoma unless we understand that it is a question of the etheric body playing a dominant role, and that this dominance is not brought under control and broken down by appropriate action on the part of the astral body and the ego organization.

In the first case therefore the physical body is given full rein, as it were; it resists the etheric body and proliferates without restraint to produce the tumour. In the second case proliferation is said to be caused by an overweening domineering etheric body.

I should like to try to resolve this apparent contradiction. To begin with, the healthy, normal etheric body and its functions will be called to mind, after which I intend to consider abnormalities in the etheric body, and finally move on to discuss therapy. Rudolf Steiner said the following about carcinoma:

> It is evident from this that if the etheric body is properly understood a way opens up by which full insight may gradually be gained into one of the worst diseases to befall the human race, and treatment may be guided in the right direction as we come to understand the non-physical actions of medicines. In this particular case we must look to the etheric body if we wish to gain real understanding of the disease.

The birth of the etheric body occurred during the Sun stage of our earth and was the gift of exalted spirits – the Kyriotetes, Dynamis and Exusiai. It is the Exusiai, or Spirits of Form, in particular who accompany the human race through all stages of development, endowing human beings with their constituent principles. During the Sun stage they gave their etheric body in sacrifice, the Kyriotetes let this gift of light flow through the physical body, refining it, and the Dynamis caused regular currents to develop within it, currents that the Exusiai in turn made into forms that would have a certain permanence. We must visualize this ancient Sun time of the earth as a world of magical beauty, when the very earliest human forms, created out of warmth and endowed with ether, started to flower in glowing colours.

During the Ancient Moon stage of the earth that was to follow, the subtly physical nature of those early seeds of men who were slowly awakening to conscious awareness, came to be increasingly organized into human form as they listened to the music of the spheres, and as evolution progressed. The human etheric body finally came to be differentiated into warmth, light, sound and life ether. With this, the archetypal image of our etheric body had been born. The spirit soul of man, grown independent and indi-vidual since, can use this archetype as a model when it descends into incarnation, to form its etheric garment. With the help of the hierarchies, the spirit soul passing through the Moon sphere draws on all the powers of the planetary system to shape the etheric form that envelops it, an experience which Rudolf Steiner has put most beautifully into words:

> Sprung forth from the cosmos, a form of light,
> Grown to strength through Sun, in the realm where Moon holds sway,
> You are endowed by Mars in sonance creative,
> And by Mercury's swift to-and-fro, setting limbs in motion,

> Illumined you are with Jupiter's radiant
>   wisdom
> And by Venus in beauty that comes
>   bearing love,
> That Saturn, the ancient of worlds, in
>   inwardness of spirit
> May commit you to be extant in space
>   and evolve in time.

This individually-fashioned star-etheric body, the image of the cosmos in which the whole sky is reflected, gradually becomes an integral part of the physical body during the first two seven-year periods of life, replacing the etheric body we have inherited from our parents. Up to the seventh year, a clairvoyant looking at a little child is still able to see this etheric cosmos. After this it contracts in the region of the heart, replacing the 'rotting' etheric body of the heart that the child had inherited. Once sexual maturity has been reached, everything we do feel and think, the actions of the astral body and the ego, are inscribed upon this heart cosmos. After death the heart will finally expand again into a cosmic sphere, handing over the fruits of our earth life to the cosmic spirits with whom we will then work together to determine our next karma.

Rudolf Steiner described the etheric body as a kind of doppelganger of the physical body, though it had buoyancy where the other had gravity, and a centrifugal tendency as opposed to the centripetal tendency of the physical. Its basic colour, he said, was like the colour of fresh peach blossom. The etheric body has something of a centre in the region of the heart, and this etheric heart is a marvellous organ shimmering in all colours, from which currents stream to all other parts of the body.

Every night, when the ego and astral body depart from the living human body, exalted spirits are working on the constituent principles that remain lying in bed. The physical products of effort that cause the body to feel tired are removed, so that the etheric body can fully irradiate it. We experience this as the miracle of renewal, of feeling fresh again, when we wake up. We can see that the etheric body is the vehicle of spiritual light for the astral body and ego; it is the Christophorus, the archetype of health.

The etheric body works not only on the physical body, of course. As the physical body gradually comes to be fully developed, the etheric body is able to separate from it in stages and become the basis on which the ability to think, to form mental images and to remember can develop. We see the same laws pertaining to thought as to growth, namely, metamorphosis and reproduction. One thought follows another, just as in the plant, where etheric activity is most clearly manifest, leaf follows leaf. And just as metamorphosis causes the transformation of the basic leaf form into many different and more complex forms in the plant, so a simple initial thought can evolve into the rich fabric of a tissue of thought. Thoughts, too, can be reproduced, and interaction between two thoughts can give rise to a third. On the other hand there are also thoughts that kindle a flame in us, and these arise in the thinking process as the purely spiritual elements of Inspiration and of Intuition come in; they are like the flowers of a plant that arise due to an astral impulse.

Not being clairvoyant we are unable to perceive the etheric body directly, but we can gain sensitive awareness of it. Look at a baby, for instance, as it lies asleep – healthy, pink-cheeked and chubby. There you have the etheric almost tangibly before you. A properly functioning etheric body bases itself on the fluid organism; it is the constituent principle that comes to expression in the gentle flow of body fluids, in the turgor of the skin, in the rosy colour of incarnation, and also in good hair growth, rapid healing of wounds, endurance and rapid recovery. Other aspects are logical sequence of thought, a good memory, and the ability to visualize things. Loving observation regularly practised can thus help us to get a feeling for the etheric body, and this will of its own accord bring fluidity, a certain mobility into our thought processes. With healing in any form we, as physicians, always have to address ourselves in differentiated fashion to this particular principle.

Today, however, this gift of the gods, this light-filled life body in its rich play of colour, resonant and warm, is facing certain serious threats.

When in the far distant past of earth evolution the Moon separated from the earth under the guidance of Jehovah, to free the earth from hardening tendencies and enable it to develop, certain ahrimanic spirits remained behind and unlawfully built their fastnesses in the earthy, watery element below the surface of the earth. These backward Moon powers are active in ebb and flood, in volcanic features and in earthquakes. They also come to expression in gravity and magnetism. In human physiology, they influence our unconscious metabolic functions, beleaguering us every night as we lie asleep. This was less marked in earlier times, but in the present age people are more and more delivered into the hands of these demonic powers. They approach the human spirit soul, that is, the ego and astral body, deceiving it by presenting evil as good and good as evil. We return to waking consciousness with these powers of evil temptation inside us, and the spirit soul, grown amoral during the night, only takes in moral impulses again as it enters into the physical and etheric bodies, for these are the bearers of religious and moral principles.

We can so easily see it in ourselves, how we go to sleep at night full of the best intentions and these seem to have been wiped out when we wake up in the morning. We are only able to revive them again once we are fully incarnated, something that takes longer with some people than it does with others.

On the other hand there are particularly good people whose moral sense imprints itself so deeply on the spirit soul during the day that they cannot enter the spiritual world in an amoral state. You will find that they have problems sleeping, their consciences being so sensitive that even minor faults are taken as evil and become a torment. Criminals on the other hand are said to sleep particularly soundly (there is statistical evidence for this), not having developed a moral conscience. They will therefore feel great satisfaction on hearing Ahriman's insinuations, for he is confirming their view that evil is good. Do not be too unhappy, therefore, if you have problems sleeping. It should be noted, however, that not every good sleeper is a criminal.

The ahrimanic powers, Moon powers that have stayed behind and become retarded –

there are Venus spirits of the same ilk –
also have a go at the etheric body which
stays behind when we are asleep. Their life
element is the Old Moon ether, which we may
also call the Earth ether, that comes to
expression in formless proliferation and is
the opposite of the cosmic ether from which
our etheric body took its individual form.
Every night, these powers try to give the
human being an etheric body made of Earth
ether, to infiltrate his Sun etheric body with
the earthly Moon ether. They succeed only
very rarely in this project which aims to
make human beings into etheric ghosts after
death and in this way to conserve the earth,
preventing it from becoming spiritual and
entering into the Jupiter state. But (and here
we come to the heart of the matter) although
demons only very rarely achieve their aim of
infiltrating the whole human etheric body
with Earth ether, they nevertheless manage
frequently to introduce the laws of the Earth
ether, the proliferative powers of the Ancient
Moon, into the normal etheric body, and
these then cause diseases in the physical
body.

It will not be difficult to guess which
diseases these are. They are the diseases
arising not from external causes but from
inside. Rudolf Steiner enumerated them: all
kinds of tumours, carcinomas, and also
metabolic diseases, above all diabetes.

Ahriman may thus win partial victories,
but these also spell his doom. Because the
physical nature of human beings is at times
ruined by disease, the ahrimanic powers are
no longer able to take hold of the aspect of
the human being that is characterized by the
instincts and drives that arise from the
metabolic region – which is another goal they

are pursuing. The sub-human drives and passions are put 'in check' by the disease, and particularly by cancer in its advanced stages, and are then no longer any good to the ahrimanic powers in their desire to build up a sub-human population. Thus illness is fundamentally an act of grace from the world of the spirit, the only means the good spirits have of saving humanity from the clutches of Ahriman.

That is how Rudolf Steiner described it. And we can see how our etheric body is night after night exposed to the danger of being obscured, ahrimanized, and we may assume that the risk is particularly great for the parts of the etheric body that are not irradiated, structurally organized and fully governed by the higher principles. Thus we can visualize, for instance, that the etheric powers of childhood, which ought to metamorphose into powers of thought and the ability to form mental images at certain stages in life, can remain in the physical organism and form islands within it, as it were, if the child's upbringing has not been right. Tumours developing in later life may originate in such enclosures, which may be present in any organ and consist of an excess of organizing vitality. Such an etheric island has dropped out of an otherwise well-organized etheric body and becomes a welcome prey for Ahriman, who can infiltrate his proliferative Earth ether here.

The same applies when the etheric body predominates in some organ or other where the ego and astral body are not in full control, a situation I have already referred to. This again is a point where the Earth-Moon ether can invade, because that part of the etheric is not fully structured by the higher principles. Rudolf Steiner has given an exact description of the dynamics of the constituent principles in carcinogenesis (the development of cancer). He often compared a carcinoma in its beginning stages to a sense organ in the wrong place, and particularly to an ear-like configuration. In a muscle, for instance, all four principles are intimately interrelated. In the eye on the other hand, the upper two, the ego and the astral body, separate from the lower two, the etheric body and the physical body. In the ear, the bonds between ego and astral body on the one hand and the etheric and physical bodies on the other are also loosened. When a tumour develops, therefore, the constituent principles fall apart, leaving the door wide open for proliferative powers.

It is also possible to imagine that in so-called 'cancer houses', (i.e. where beds are positioned in places where there is a concentration of geodetic lines, and earth radiation, also called electromagnetic radiation, streams upwards as if through holes in the surface of the earth) the proliferative powers of Ancient Moon ethers may come through with particular force.

That is how I would explain the apparent contradiction to which I drew attention at the beginning. A hypertrophic, overweening etheric body or isolated ether islands are abnormalities compared with a healthy etheric body. If they are brought into the domain of the Earth ether, if the organs concerned are infiltrated with proliferative principles, the consequence will be 'rebellion' of the physical powers in that part against the normal etheric powers of the body, with the etheric body no longer able to reach this foreign construct which has arisen from sources outside the human being and is now following its own laws. Ether islands and dominance of the etheric body are more the initial stages in the cancer process. The withdrawal of the etheric body as it puts a distance between itself and the proliferation of foreign etheric principles represents an advanced stage. As the cancer process advances and secondary tumours develop, more and more parts of the normal etheric body are alienated from it, until the etheric body finally collapses and cachexia (extreme emaciation) develops.

It should also be clear from the above that carcinogenesis can take many forms and that it shows individual differences. The weak spots in the human etheric and physical bodies that have been mentioned may have their origin in previous earth lives. Carcinogenic elements in the sphere of the astral body and the ego are predisposing mental states and these, too, may have been influenced by karmic conditions. Finally there are the vast numbers of external carcinogens.

I have deliberately concentrated on the etheric body so far, and now want to go on to consider treatment. We have looked at the way in which the constituent principles dissociate as cancer develops. The powers of mistletoe are the exact opposite of this, and the plant therefore provides a medium that can be used to treat the root causes. Rudolf Steiner put this very clearly in his last medical lecture, which he gave in London in 1924:

Mistletoe acts as a substance from the outside world that addresses itself to the proliferating ether substance in the carcin-

> oma, and by pushing back physical substance enhances the action of the astral body, thus causing the tumour to crumble and collapse upon itself.

A year earlier he had said:

> If the etheric body comes into effect in the right way, being first of all fully organized by the ego and astral body . . we are supporting a healing process that wants to be there, the human organization being what it is.

So you see that mistletoe is capable of reversing the process in which the constituent principle is dissociated. It is able to do so because it is itself related to the Ancient Moon powers, and indeed still grows on the Ancient Moon today, for the trunks and branches of trees are atavistic remnants from the earlier Moon state of the earth.

Every plant develops on the basis of two vital currents. One of these is the 'wood sap', as it is called; it rises from the earthy fluid sphere of the Ancient Moon region beneath the surface of the earth and forms the trunks and branches of trees, drying up soon after this. The other current that comes to meet it is the 'life sap' from the region of fluid in air that is peripheral to the earth. This comes from above to enliven the plant and circulates within it, producing leaves, buds and flowers. The wood sap corresponds to the cellular fluid in humans, for in cells, too, the proliferative tendency of the Ancient Moon is at work, threatening to chain human beings to the earth unless the organizing powers of the higher principles establish form and differentiation. Those powers are active in the blood, and they correspond to the life sap in plants that comes from the cosmic powers of the periphery.

The mistletoe absorbs the Moon-earth ether, but then, being very much a light-seeking plant, turns to the periphery, and through this affinity to light is able to overcome the proliferative tendency within itself. This helps us to understand Rudolf Steiner's statement, already quoted, which I offer once again:

> Mistletoe acts as a substance from the outside world that addresses itself to the proliferating ether substance in the carci-noma, and by pushing back physical substance enhances the action of the astral body, thus causing the tumour to crumble and collapse upon itself.

What can we do to support the etheric body, this most important principle, in the fight against cancer, protecting it against the corruption that demonic powers threaten to impose on it night after night? There are many possibilities, just a few of which are given below.

We can strengthen the etheric body medi-cally. The first choice for this would be gold, *Aurum*, for this harmonizes the whole organism from the heart. Rudolf Steiner called it the 'vitalizer'. We may also use the power that lies in hawthorn, *Prunus spinosa*, a plant that conserves its vital powers, being slow-growing and liable to contract into thorns, until it finally lets them enter into the sweet astringent fruits in autumn. In a similar way, lemon used in baths will hold together the patient's vital powers that threaten to ebb away, and in this way strengthen the etheric body.

Taken in physical amounts, these substances do not, fundamentally, have a direct action. They relate the human being to the healing elemental spirits at night, and this relationship develops health-giving potential when we are awake.

We are however also able to influence the etheric body directly, mainly by paying careful attention to the sleep life of cancer patients. A number of drugs are available that will help them to sleep, among them *Avena sativa* (oat), *Passiflora* (passion flower) and *Conchae* (oyster shell, natural calcium carbonate). Phosphorus 5x in the mornings and Phosphorus 30 at night (5x and 30 refer to homeopathic potencies) may be used to regulate the day and night rhythm. In remedial eurythmy, the Hallelujah exercise and the 'A' (as in father), walking backwards, will often prove marvellously effective. According to Rudolf Steiner, however, we should not seek to achieve sleep at all costs with cancer patients. It is better not to sleep for a time rather than induce sleep with chemical sleeping drugs and give free access to the ahrimanic spirits. Extremes should of course be avoided, for a patient who is endlessly awake may well become so low and nervous that one of the more powerful sleeping drugs will have to be used now and again, to enable that patient to enter into the world of the spirit. Combination with *Aurum* 10x, for example, will afford a certain protection in this case.

Carefully chosen artistic activities during the day will make it possible for patients to have encounters with the protective spirits of higher hierarchies who channel vitalizing forces towards the etheric body. When the right way of speaking is practised in creative speech, for instance, the whole of the human being is involved, but particularly the etheric and astral bodies. When language has been consciously cultivated, the spiritual content of it will continue to resonate and allow us to communicate with the world of the angels at night, who will be well pleased at this.

Someone who neglects the artistic potential of language, using it merely as a means of communication, is in a state of torment at night, able to see spiritual entities but unable to communicate with them, unable to hear the World Word that they speak. Rudolf Steiner described how the brain is then filled with the racket, the physical murmuring, the scraping, grinding, rolling and brushing noises of the mineral world at night, and also how the racket, the hissing, sighing, rushing, knocking, drip-dripping noises of the vegetable world influence the circulation. The higher worlds are no longer able to come in and establish a configuration in this case, and the human being comes out of his sleep with a dreadful feeling that there is something lacking.

Eurythmy can also be a tremendous help. It makes us experience the spiritual nature of arms and hands, so that we do not merely use them as tools but sense the sublime spiritual nature of the etheric aspect of these limbs that link us, from the heart, with the regions of the stars.

The cultivation of proper sleep may also be supported by clay-modelling, to strengthen the patient's own etheric body, by painting, to give a conscious experience of colour qualities, and by light and colour therapy, where looking, listening, speaking and touching are practised in rhythmical alternation, to make the patient fully part again of the seven planetary spheres of the etheric world.

The etheric body is also strengthened by listening to single notes, as recommended by Rudolf Steiner. The rich abundance of feeling that can be experienced in a melody must be carefully trained by working with single notes, making it possible to experience their rich content with the same intensity as when listening to a melody.

With this, we are already beginning to act on the etheric body via the astral body. It is possible to intensify the effect by encouraging patients to develop a conscious relationship to the kingdoms of nature. We may suggest to them that they should look at and enjoy the beautiful colours and forms of the mineral world. To enter into pure observation of a plant, following its growth, its metamorphoses, has healing qualities. The gestures of an animal can also be observed, letting us experience the instinctual world that lies behind them. Such exercises will help patients to establish the right relation-ship to the elemental spirits in these kingdoms. At night they will then experience, though unconsciously, the flowing interplay of colours, the living world of sound, and achieve the right relationship to the Archai, the spirits of Personal Individuality. The Archai help us to let the astral body enter properly into the etheric body. But they will also help us to go to sleep properly. This will give rise to that aura, or atmosphere, as Rudolf Steiner put it, through which human beings are able to take a proper hold of their etheric and physical bodies on waking in the morning, and to let them go again at night, trusting in the spirits.

The etheric body is in constant flow of thought, even when we are not consciously thinking. Conscious thought is merely a reflection of this flow. Conscious, ego-guided thinking does however have a purifying power that has its effect on the astral and etheric bodies. Thus the doppelganger of Johannes Thomasius in the mystery play says·

> Johannes had to keep apart
> From Maria during life.
> Since then he has given himself to
>   rigorous thought;
> And this has powers that purify the
>   soul.
> What then arose from the purity of
>   his thinking
> Has also poured into me; I changed;
> I sense his purity within myself.

Thus we must try, for example, to get our patients to think clearly with the aid of Rudolf Steiner's *Philosophy of Freedom*, however hard this may seem. One way is to get them to read a paragraph each morning and then write down what they have read in their own words. This, by the way, is also a good method of regulating digestive function, the bowels. Thinking and intestinal activity are intimately bound up with each other.

The purifying power of clear thinking has an effect on the astral body and therefore on the unconscious drives and passions which the ahrimanic powers approach at night with the intention of creating a subterranean race of demons. This purifying power will make them shrink back.

The centre of the etheric body, its heart and focal point, can be very consciously influenced via the ego by practising six basic exercises: 1, controlling our thoughts; 2, logical consistency in our actions; 3, perseverance; 4, tolerance; 5, an open mind towards the phenomena of life – faith, trust; 6, equanimity. This will irradiate and strengthen the etheric body and define its boundaries more clearly, so that the nocturnal attacks of demons are repelled. We can also strengthen the etheric body through the ego by going through the day's events backwards at night, and with any other concept that is gone through in reverse.

Finally we should try and in some way or other bring religious feeling to the patient. Let me remind you of the beautiful way in which Rudolf Steiner described this in his lecture entitled 'The Etherization of the Blood.'

When we are awake, a thought-like etheric stream is constantly rising from the blood in the region of the heart and ascending to the head, letting radiant light play around the pineal gland. During sleep, on the other hand, will impulses of a moral nature are streaming from the macrocosm through the head and to the heart. These streams are dependent on the moral qualities of the individual and a clairvoyant will perceive them in appropriate colours. If we join ourselves to Christ in our hearts, the etheric power of the blood of Christ that has streamed down into the earth and has been present in the etheric body of the earth from the time of Golgotha, can join with the thought stream as we wake up and inwardly build us up. The consequence will be that the night-time stream of will impulses coming from exalted spirits in the cosmos flows into us unimpeded, shielding us from the promptings of Ahriman. By consciously joining ourselves to Christ it is also possible to begin to develop a basis for the ability to see Him in His etheric form. He opposes the powers that are slowly destroying the earth – electricity, magnetism and nuclear power – and brings constructive powers into human civilization and culture.

There are thus many different ways of treating the etheric body in order to prevent illness and achieve healing. And there is great wisdom in the way the etheric body is differentiated. In the head, imbued with warmth, it is the light ether, enabling thought. In the middle part of the human being, it is the sound ether, through which feeling arises. In the lower human being it is the life ether, and will impulses arise from this.

By working at a higher level than that of the more unconscious actions of drugs, we are able to strengthen and support the etheric body and give it greater differentiation with artistic and religious activity, and finally also with wholly conscious egoic activity.

An attempt has been made in this paper to take up the indications given by Rudolf Steiner and look for ways and means of strengthening the etheric body to combat not only cancer but also the cancerous disease that is affecting the whole of our civilization, growing more and more threatening. The threat arising for the whole of mankind as ahrimanic and luciferic spirits are fighting both over and within the human being is indeed tremendous. It is hoped that the suggestions that have been made will encourage others to see the dangers that are arising for the etheric body, the light-breathing principle that has sprung from the cosmos, and to take steps to meet those dangers.

True healing is more than prescribing medicines, it makes it our duty to help patients to grow to health from their illness and into being new persons. How this is to be achieved in the individual case must be left to our capacity as physicians to enter into the mind and situation of a patient, to our Intuition, and to the heart we have for the healing task.

CHAPTER 3

SACRIFICE AND HEALING

Healing is a very comprehensive function, encompassing development, education and the attainment of health. I should therefore like to consider – as an archetype, as it were, of all healing – the great sacrifices that have been made to take human beings to their present stage of development.

Let us try to visualize the ancient Lemurian epoch of the earth, a kind of recapitulation of the Moon stage. First the Sun separated from the earth, then the Moon, too, departed, and Sun and Moon were now acting on the earth from outside. The earth was still watery, except for occasional islands of firmer soil. This was the time when the first man and woman to incarnate, Adam and Eve, fell into sin, but part of Adam's soul was held back and did not incarnate. This soul had all the wisdom gained from experience during the Saturn, Sun and Moon epochs, and all the love of which a human soul would be capable. It remained innocent, did not descend into incarnation, and was perceived only by initiates in their mysteries. This angelic soul experienced all the growing pains of the developing human race, of human beings who fundamentally were her brothers and sisters. The Fall had opened up the physical senses of human beings. But the onrush of sense impressions was pulling people hither and thither, tearing them apart in overwhelming sympathy and antipathy. The sister soul of

Adam dwelling in cosmic heights felt this distress and resolved to give herself up to the highest Sun spirit, to Christ, and let Him enter fully into her. Picture how this soul moved down from the crystal heaven into the region of the zodiac and you will understand how thanks to this deed the human race gained the power to stand upright and as a result was then able to put sense impressions at a distance.

Then at the beginning of the Atlantean epoch, mankind, still almost without speech at that time, found new torments arising in the course of development. Thanks to the powers of the seven planets circling the earth, human beings now had internal organs, vital organs. But these organs aroused tremendous hungers in them, or terrible disgust. And again the soul of Adam took pity, and filled with the Christ came down in descending spirals through the sphere of the planets. This transformed the effects that the planetary spirits had on the world, creating the power of moderation which established harmony between the organs. Early Atlantean man, who until then had been able to express himself only in animal sounds, became able to give expression not only to subjective but also objective contents with the beginnings of a language that probably consisted largely of vowel sounds.

We now come to the later Atlantean epoch. Human beings were now able to cope with the impressions that came through the physical sense organs, and their vital organs no longer put them under compulsion, for harmony had been created in the living physical body. However, adverse powers caused them to end up in a chaos of soul powers, with the result that people were raving, demonic, and in a certain sense also showed hypertrophy of thinking. The equilibrium between Sun and Moon activities on earth had been upset. Once again the soul of Adam sacrificed herself and, circling the earth within the Moon sphere, called upon Christ to come down, join Himself to her, and help to tame and overcome the dragon in the soul of man. A victory was won that gave rise to wisdom and consequently the ability to develop language fully as a means of communication. The human soul found harmony in the music of the spheres.

Finally, in the middle of the post-Atlantean epoch, at the turning point of time, the fourth and greatest sacrifice was called for. The human race, formerly guided by the gods, had increasingly become separated from them and entered into purely earthly consciousness. The vital powers of the earth and of man were threatening to atrophy. Disease, epidemics and misery of mind and spirit reigned on an earth that was withdrawing from the gods. At that time Christ, the great Sun Spirit who had been approaching the earth through centuries, took compassion. Yet His sacrifice was possible only because in the meantime the soul of Adam had found a body in which it could incarnate, the Nathan Jesus. The most significant spiritual streams in human history had come together to make him the vessel for the Sun God, who after three years of working as a healer had to endure and accomplish great suffering, death and the overcoming of death.

With this great sacrifice, through the Mystery of Golgotha, new life poured into the earth, the first beginnings of a future when it would become Sun, and ego power was now able to fill the constituent principles of the human being with its radiance, so that human beings awoke to independent thought.

We see from these truly wonderful events that a mysterious process forms the background to healing activity: Need and pain have to be recognized, this recognition must be transformed into compassion, a sharing of pain, and then willing surrender on one side must open up to the giving, creative stream coming from the other. The meeting of the two mysteriously gives rise to healing powers, a strength welling forth in which the sufferers, the patients, can gain new health.

During the aeons in which the archetypal healing process developed, condensing at rhythmical intervals in the four sacrifices, Christ the Sun Spirit needed helpers who would work with Him and both continue and complement His work. The Mercury spirit was the one particularly chosen for this task by Christ, a mighty spirit who, after the separation of the Sun, had shaped the planet Mercury to be his dwelling place. Healing powers are constantly issuing from this planet to this day. As Rudolf Steiner told us: 'The earth would proliferate, producing life forms all the time, carcinomas all the time, if a process were not set in opposition to this from outside the earth, from Mercury.' The function of the Mercury powers is to maintain balance, and healing of course means to restore the balance. Rudolf Steiner further said that not only would the earth proliferate, but every substance capable of forming drops would become a living form, and the metabolic region of man, where cell life predominates, would also proliferate, unless this excess of life were held in check by the planetary influence of Mercury. You see how this Mercury action plays a very particular role in the cancer process.

Mercury powers establish the balance between light and gravity, between what is above the earth and on the earth, between anabolism and catabolism, between life and death. There is an old Rosicrucian saying: 'I bear Mercury within me, who holds together Sun and Moon.' Mercury was revered as the spirit that formed the link between heaven and earth, the one to reveal human destiny. The lung as the organ representative of Mercury also acts in this way. In respiration it holds us in suspended balance between incarnation and excarnation, buoyancy and gravity. The breathing process enlivens us as we inhale oxygen, giving the used material back to the environment with the carbon dioxide. The ego began to enter with the breath in the far distant past, and it still enters with the first breath today and leaves with the last. The breath is the healer who is always with us. The E sound in Mercury reveals the human being as an individual person, it is the human being active in the 'to-and-fro of limbs set in motion.'

From the Mercury region, exalted Fire Spirits, Archangeloi, descended to earth during the Atlantean epoch to help Christ, endowing the most advanced human beings with soul and spirit and acting as the teachers of the young human race in the mystery sites, the oracles. During the day they appeared in human form to the Atlanteans, who were still partly in a dream state; at night they were seen as radiant sublime spirits. They were the priest kings of ancient Atlantis, conveying the mysteries of the universe, so that the germinating ego would gradually be able to take hold of the principles that enveloped it.

We can see their continuing activities in the great leaders of civilization during the Post-Atlantean epoch – the Rishis of India, Zarathustra during the Persian epoch, Hermes Trismegistus in ancient Egypt. It was during the Egyptian epoch that medical activity as such began in the mysteries of Mercury, where the secrets of Sun and Moon were revealed. This was where the Temple Sleep was first practised as a healing mystery, with the patients well prepared with medicaments and ritual purification before the priests introduced etheric figures into their sleep, divine figures connected with the healing principle. Among these figures it was particularly the image of Isis that related to the art of healing and helped to harmonize the constituent principles that had fallen into disorder in the disease process.

In the Greek mysteries, in Epidaurus for instance, Asclepios was performing a similar function. He was a son of Apollo, the god also revered as one who brought healing, because the playing of his lyre created harmony between thinking, feeling and will activity. In the Temple Sleep, the demigod Asclepios placed the undistorted and intact image of original man before the mind's eye, so that on waking it would irradiate the etheric body and bring about healing.

The Hermes of the Greeks, known as Mercury to the Romans, did not act directly as a medical healer, but his 'mercurial' activity embodied certain functions of the archetypal Mercury principles. Being the son of Zeus and Maya, he was the god of safe conduct, directing the paths of destiny and, as Psychopompos, guiding the soul to Hades. On winged feet he moved swiftly hither and thither, binding and loosing, and he was able to use his magic caduceus to put people to sleep and give them dreams. In his Hermes Logios aspect he bestowed the gift of the word, of eloquence. Happy events and profits made were due to him, and he was therefore also the god of merchants and thieves, particularly as he had stolen cattle from his brother Apollo when still in the cradle, innocently snuggling down again among the blankets. He is a somewhat superficial but certainly very likeable projection of the exalted Mercury spirit.

Returning to the stream of real healers, we see how the teaching function of the Fire Spirits of Mercury in the service of mankind's development gradually condensed to become healing in the medical sense. We may visualize these archangels of Mercury as having physical existence in fire and wind. This is expressed in Psalm 104: 'Who makest the wind thy messengers and flames of fire thy servants.' This image also relates to Woden who became an emissary of Mercury in Egyptian times and was sent to be the teacher of the Nordic mysteries. He was seen to hold sway in the World Wind, with his breath creating language, wisdom coming to living expression in sound. The elements were his kingdom, and he also guided the destinies of war and of death. At a later time, this same Mercury spirit, Woden, appeared as the spirit that illumined the Indian prince Gautama, uniting himself with him and elevating him to Buddha status when he was in his 29th year. The working of this Mercury spirit, which in the North had been more macrocosmic, manifesting in outward

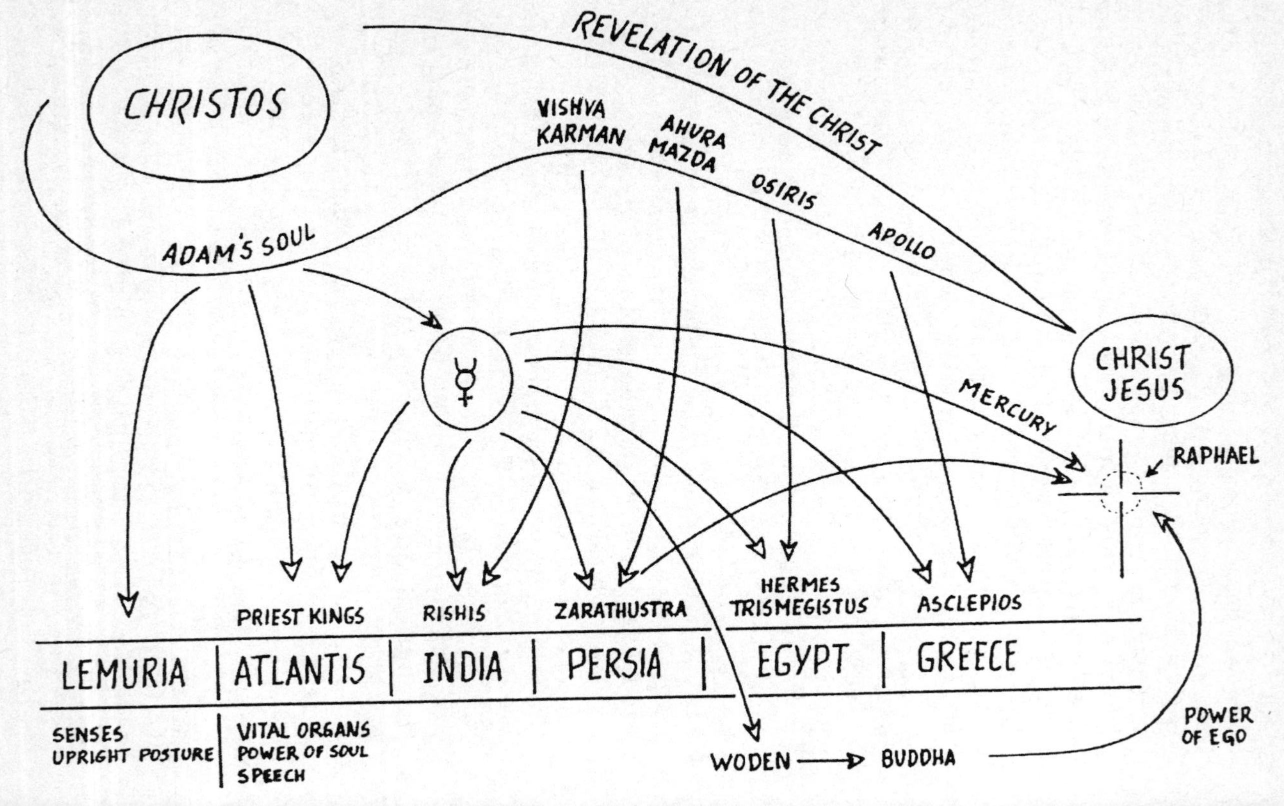
CHRISTOS
REVELATION OF THE CHRIST
VISHVA KARMAN
AHURA MAZDA
OSIRIS
APOLLO
CHRIST JESUS
ADAM'S SOUL
MERCURY
RAPHAEL
PRIEST KINGS
RISHIS
ZARATHUSTRA
HERMES TRISMEGISTUS
ASCLEPIOS
LEMURIA | ATLANTIS | INDIA | PERSIA | EGYPT | GREECE
SENSES
UPRIGHT POSTURE
VITAL ORGANS
POWER OF SOUL
SPEECH
WODEN ——→ BUDDHA
POWER OF EGO

ways, then became an entirely inward process in the teaching of compassion and love, preparing the powers of the human soul for their highest development. We can visualize how Sleipnir, the eight-footed horse who bore Woden through the clouds, became transformed into the eightfold path of inner development shown by the Buddha.

We are now approaching the turning point of time. The Christ spirit had gradually come closer to the earth during the Post-Atlantean epoch, revealing himself as Vishva Karman in ancient India, Ahura Mazda to the Persians, Osiris to the Egyptians, Apollo to the Greeks. He was always accompanied by the pure soul of man that had not yet become incarnate. Now, at the turning point of time, the sublime Sun god had completed his descent. At this pivotal point in world evolution all the streams met: the Sun stream of Christ Jesus and the representatives of the Mercury stream. The soul body of the Buddha as Nirmanakaya poured his glory upon the Nathan Jesus child, and the Zarathustra spirit united with the child in his twelfth year. Then, at the end of His sojourn on earth, one can gain the impression that the highest Mercury spirit himself, having until then sent only his emissaries to mankind, united himself with Christ. In the Mystery of Golgotha, Christ became the true Mercury, *Christus verus Mercurius.* One feels that silent reverence is the only way in which we can contemplate the sheer magnitude of this event.

But we must also try to understand the significance which this event holds for us today and for the future.

Christ had now united with the earth. The aura of His Spirit enveloped it, filling it with radiance, and all the hierarchies now knew: a new age has begun for the earth, the Mars age has given way to the Mercury age. Christ then moved through all the occult schools, and the spiritual leaders of the human race bowed before his majesty. The one, however, who had been his helper from time immemorial, the highest Mercury spirit who was now united and ruling with Him, became transformed into Raphael. The fire of Christ's love transformed the caduceus with its serpents into a rod of flame. Every spring, Raphael brings the Christ principle into the elements with this rod, transforming them into healing powers. Every autumn, Raphael stands by the side of man 'his mind inclined to every breath taken,' bestowing healing powers on the human rhythmical system. Raphael thus is the healing aspect, as it were, of Christ's work in the periphery, a work that brings blessing to souls in the cosmic rhythms.

Paul was the first to see the Vanquisher of Death, the Risen One, in the etheric world. Destiny then brought him a disciple who became his friend and physician: Luke, the Greek. In an earlier life, Luke had gone through the Bull initiation, achieving full control of the instinctual life. In this life he had become a great physician who was even capable of rousing the dead. In a restless, lonely, searching life, he finally found the one he had been longing to meet ever since he was a young man, the 'Unknown', the 'God to Come' of the Greeks, the Christ. During the time when he and Paul spread Christianity in the world, he grew and matured to become the first Christian physician. If you study his gospel today, you can sense how its words come from the etheric realm of the Risen One, and that within them lie powers of healing and of resurrection. It is not for nothing that Rudolf Steiner put particular emphasis on the need to study this gospel when he was speaking to young doctors.

> Far, far my soul reaches out, to praise thee, Lord of Life; jubilant, my spirit rejoices in thee, divine bringer of salvation . . .

The beginning of this Mercury age in which we now are may well coincide with the deepest descent of healing impulses into out-and-out materialism, yet the rosy dawn of healing in the spirit of Christ that can be experienced in Luke and his gospel is still there, it is still alive. Noticed by just a few, it became transformed into a stream of light from which emerged, like stars in the firmament of heaven, the teachers of Chartres, the guardians of the Grail, the Templars, and the Rosicrucians, to mention just a few.

Today we are at the beginning of a new phase in the Mercury age, a time when as physicians we are called upon to join in making the utmost effort, particularly in our struggle to heal cancer.

Let us once more consider the archetypal healing process in the four Deeds of Christ: Blazing forth from it is the spiritual law according to which two must always work together if a third principle is to arise as something new. Dr Ita Wegman, a physician deeply imbued with the will to heal, apoproached Rudolf Steiner in this century, the century of Christ's embodiment in etheric form, with the quest for new healing mysteries. Rudolf Steiner revealed to us, and to all who are engaged in healing work, the path we have to follow to become true Christian healers in a world where medical work has become the computer-aided repairing of individual parts, leaving aside consideration of the human being as a whole.

I should like to conclude by giving you an outline of this three-stage path. It is a path that with suitable variation can also be followed by anyone who in some form or other wants to take part in the work of healing the phenomena of our time. First of all it is essential to be fully conversant with present-day knowledge, however dry it may seem. To take the bull by the horns was one of the maxims in Rudolf Steiner's life. We must not shrink from struggling through the abstract concepts of modern science, and enter into Ahriman's sphere with courage and in full awareness. To accomplish this, we shall however need the utterly dedicated will to heal that arises out of compassion and love. This, then, is the first prerequisite.

The first stage of the path takes us from a knowledge of the kingdoms of nature and of the four constituent principles of the human being into the world of the elements: earth, water, air, and fire. We must enter into these with mind and heart, so that they can truly be experienced and come to life in us when any aspect of nature is studied. This will also mean that the constituent principles become not a rigid system but living experience. You will experience how the dead rocks of our mountain ranges are akin to our skeletal system, the foundations of our physical form. In the life-giving springs, streams and rivers, we can experience something of the swelling, burgeoning quality of our own etheric body. And are not the gales that drive the scudding clouds comparable to certain soul states? When the sun finally rises above the horizon flaming in victory, we can come to experience something of the power of the ego in this picture.

In the second stage we enter more deeply into esoteric realms with the mantrams Rudolf Steiner has given in his course of lectures for young doctors. It is a difficult path, but a fruitful one, taking us from insight gained into the working of elemental spirits within the kingdoms of nature to the sphere of planetary powers and the influences of the zodiac. Now the whole of nature and man himself become the essential expression of a divine world order that lives in rhythms. Regularly carried out, such exercises will create a relationship between our astral bodies and the healing spirits whom we encounter in the periphery during the night. In the morning, we may then experience how the urge to give help grows stronger all the time, thanks to these night-time encounters.

The last and most difficult stage challenges us to develop moral qualities through three renunciations: First, none of the things we have so far worked for and achieved must be misused to give power. A physician who is in a position of power is no longer a physician. Anyone capable of healing illness is also capable of producing it. Woe betide the physician who misuses this ability! Next, we will find that the medicines we have worked so hard to penetrate with our understanding will lose their effect on we ourselves the more we get to know them. As physicians, we will not respond to treatment with them. This is the second renunciation.

Finally, we must always try to forget everything we have learned so far when we are face to face with the sufferer. This is the third renunciation. We must try to take the patient's suffering into ourselves, to feel our way into it, making ourselves into a vessel for the healing word that wants to come in, through the power of Raphael-Christ and His helpers, so that the warmth element of the healing deed can unfold.

Being a physician will thus never be a matter of routine; it will constantly be imbued with new life as we listen for the healing Inspiration. The path is long and hard, and most of us are still raw beginners. But the situation in the world today urgently calls for people who are prepared to follow this path and serve healing in its fullest sense. The Mercury impulse of the present is waiting to be taken up by us.

CHAPTER 4

THE POWER OF THE HUMAN EGO:
FROM DARKNESS TO LIGHT

Imagine you are all alone, walking along an underground passage in a mine, and suddenly all the lights go out. What would this feel like? Fear and fright would no doubt be the first reaction, the fear of losing yourself in nothingness. It would need all your inner resources to hold on to yourself. If then a light were to appear suddenly in the distance, a brightness coming towards you, a liberating feeling of relief would arise and stream out towards that light.

This simple example will help us to grow inwardly attuned so that we may come to understand the tremendous words at the beginning of the Bible, the original polarity between light and darkness:

> In the beginning God created the heaven
>   and the earth.
> And the earth was without form, and
>   void;
> And darkness was upon the face of
>   the deep.
> And God said, Let there be light:
> And there was light.
> And God saw the light, that it was good:
> And God divided the light from the
>   darkness.

Describing the evolution of the world as seen in the light of spiritual science, Rudolf Steiner wrote how the Saturn age of earth evolution was one of warmth where total darkness prevailed and the consciousness of the then germinal human beings was held in the darkness of dreamless sleep. Then creation took another step and the Sun stage was reached. Here warmth condensed to air, and at the same time a great light shone forth. What a sublime event that describes. Following the birth of time on ancient Saturn, space came into being at the Sun stage. There had to be light before there could be space. On the other hand, light also produces life, and so the human etheric or life body arose in its germinal stage, and the beginnings of conscious awareness dimly appeared.

Now we may ask ourselves: Does light really call forth life and conscious awareness? What does modern science have to say about it? Well, it established the process known as photosynthesis in which water and carbon dioxide from the atmosphere enter into a sequence of complex reactions to produce carbohydrates, the building material of the plant world. The element phosphorus, the light-bearer, plays a major role in this. The whole however is only possible under the influence of light.

The plant world uses between 300 and 500 thousand million metric tons of carbon each year to build itself up in this way, liberating corresponding amounts of oxygen in the process. This provides the essential basis for the life of oxygen-breathing creatures, i.e. animals and humans. Light is therefore like a magic wand used to condense gases and fluids into living solid matter.

Light . . . what is it really? To the modern scientist light represents a tiny section of the whole spectrum of electromagnetic waves. Wave lengths range from 18,000 kilometres to fractions of a nanometre (the thousand millionth part of a metre). The alternating current used for technical purposes, to drive trams, for instance, has the longest wave lengths. The shortest waves are those of gamma radiations produced in nuclear reactions. Visible light occupies a very narrow space within the shortwave range, from 300 to 700 micrometres, i.e. millionths of a metre.

This way of looking at it reduces the 'honest light', as Rudolf Steiner called it, which streams through cosmic space to mere electricity. Anyone who has the right kind of feeling for this will however know that there is a tremendous difference between the quality of light and the quality of electricity. You can experience this yourself by exposing yourself to an electric shock and comparing this to the feeling of joy and vitality that comes with the spring sun. Think of the Easter verse from Rudolf Steiner's *Seelenkalender* (translated by Owen Barfield as *The Year Participated*, 1985):

> When out from far and wide
> The sun calls to the mind and sense of
>   man
> And joy from in the soul with light
>   grows one
> In act of contemplation . . .

'Good and evil become one blur if light is considered to be the same as electricity,' Rudolf Steiner said. Indeed he went even further: 'Electricity has got to the nerves of people in the present age. It has struck to take away anything that has to do with turning towards the spirit.' People's thoughts are entirely caught up in the web of electricity. If an atomistic view is taken of the matter, atoms become the bearers of death. If on the other hand matter is seen in terms of electricity, and with modern views that is the case, evil enters in.

So what is the reality of light? In the first course of lectures he gave to members of the medical profession, Rudolf Steiner said it was wrong to say that light came from the sun. Light is in fact invisible. Only illuminated bodies are visible. The real light originates in the etheric world, a world that surrounds the earth in differentiated spheres. It is produced in the sphere of light, which is above the sphere of warmth. There it sprouts and grows the way plants do on earth. Light does not however travel on and on into infinity; it does not vanish into infinity but only goes as far as a limiting sphere and then bounces back elastically. Its quality is different on the way back from what it was on the way out. The light radiating outward from the sphere of light ether surrounding the earth is reflected at some distance away, and the reflective element that throws back the light was seen as the sun by the ancient initiates.

Considering the difference between light and electricity we now come to an important point, which also brings us back to the human being, the real object of our deliberations.

There is a spiritual law according to which the moral impulses of human beings provide the germ, the seed, for a natural world of the future. Thus the plant world of the future Jupiter stage of our earth is already being determined now, through our moral ideals. Now if the moral principles of today are going to be the reality behind the natural world of that future planet, behind the forces of nature on Jupiter-Earth, then we may conclude that a moral element from the past must be behind the forces of nature as we know them today. Electricity, a force which has only been utilized since the eighteenth century, is such a force of nature. If we look at electricity today it represents a moral reality of the past which, however, has turned into evil. Asked the direct question as to what electricity was, Rudolf Steiner replied: 'Electricity is a sub-material form of light. Light is most severely compressed in it. It belongs to the sub-physical astral world which is governed by Lucifer, the fallen light-bearer.' Electricity may thus be regarded as the fallen brother of light. The powers that are behind the darkness on the other hand, behind the polar opposite of light, are ahrimanic.

It is however important that we learn to deal with this element which we call evil. It is a necessary part of evolution, offering resistance so that goodness may gain strength in combating it. On the other hand we must not allow the powers of adversity to overwhelm us. None of us would like to do without electric light, without oil-fired central heating, or any form of transport today. But it is important that we see these things to be what they are.

So far we have only been considering external light. In ancient times, when Christ as spirit of the universe still dwelt in the Sun and acted from there, this external light was filled with life. Today it has become mineral by nature, dead light. Yet that is the only way in which freedom is possible — that the light leaves us unmolested, as it were, and does not essentially determine our progress.

When we take up high moral ideals with enthusiasm, the impulse for this arises from the profoundest depths in the life of our will and feelings. This impulse has an effect on our body warmth organization, so that a direct link is established between soul and body. Life coming into the warmth organization, in which the ego lives, also brings warmth to the air organization, in which the astral body lives. Air always has light in it, and this impulse of warmth therefore also creates inner light. If we come aglow with moral ideas, and our ego becomes wholly active in the process, we liberate the light that is hidden in the air, and seeds of luminescence appear in the astral body.

As the process continues sounds begin to arise from source points within the fluid organization, which provides a basis for the etheric body, and finally seeds of life begin to stir in the physical body. These are all consequences of developing enthusiasm for moral ideals. The last two stages do of course occur at profoundly unconscious levels, but we are perfectly able to perceive the warmth of enthusiasm and the brightness of the light that illumines our awareness. If the ideas that enthuse us are then actually put into effect, we are able to perceive their fruitfulness. One thing that is certain is that after death we carry the impulses of warmth, light, music of the spheres and life we have produced into the cosmos, and there they play a role in the creation of the future world. Human beings are thus responsible for the future, right down to creating the material reality and shaping the natural world of future earth stages.

The situation is quite different when it comes to intellectual thoughts and theoretical ideas. These have a chilling effect on the warmth organism; they paralyse the generation of inner light. The universe dies if exposed to theoretical ideas, for such intellectual thoughts usually relate to things that have already come into being and reached completion. On the other hand, these analytical, dissecting thoughts – they may be said to offer us corpses of the universe – enable us to develop self-awareness. Dead thoughts can also give rise to enthusiasm, i.e. to thoughts full of life, if we fire them in the sphere of the will, where our moral – and immoral – impulses have their origin. Thus we really carry the passing and the coming-into-being of worlds within us, both dead and living light. Rudolf Steiner appealed to our sense of responsibility when he said in conclusion:

> If there were just a dozen people with a shining moral and spiritual enthusiasm, the earth would after all attain to the radiance of a spiritual sun; even if millions of people were to perish devoid of spirituality in an age of misery.

We are therefore standing at a point where two streams of light cross. The dead light of the external world enters into us with every breath we take and through everything we perceive with the senses. We meet it with the thinking activity that is the product of inner light generation. This activity, too, is dead. We can enliven it by consciously letting will impulses and feeling enter into our thinking. If we merely stare at the material world, registering it with the intellect – on

organized tours for instance, when impressions flood in - nothing can really come to
life. If there is to be a real enlivenment, it
will be necessary for the whole of our soul
life to come alive, following the upward
swing of inner jubilation and also the
downward swing of pain. A good exercise in
this direction is contemplative observation of
the plant world, letting life coming into
being, coming into flower, enter into our
meditation, and then in contrast with this
consider life fading away and dying. Such
meditative contemplation will also reveal the
healing powers inherent in plants. The
cosmic soul element of external light becomes
unveiled in this light that is given life from
within. The light reaching us from outside is
dead, but soul qualities are borne towards
us on the wings of light, which here is
representative of all sensory perception. If
we meet this cosmic soul element with a soul
life in which we are full human beings, if
we unfold the will in active sensory perception, we establish a relationship to outer
nature in which the Christ fire lights up.
just as it lights up when the will fires our
thoughts to create moral impulses. Future
mankind will need to be active in this way,
in what we may call the Michael culture.

The inner light process relates to the
mystery of the carbon process. We are able
to develop into human beings because animal
nature has been put outside. Through our
egoity we attain to the upright position,
through our egoity we master our soul forces,
through our egoity we also denude the food
we eat of all traces of its origin, excreting
it as a dead, mineral-like product. Animal
excretions still contain life and can therefore
be used as agricultural fertilizer. Human

beings kill the substance of the outside world completely, and also keep their intestinal fauna and flora within certain limits, using the powers of the ego organization to overcome the process of becoming animal.

Any devitalized food which is not excreted has to go through a neutral or zero point on passing the intestinal wall, i.e. it needs to be made entirely spiritual before it is transformed into human substance. This also applies to carbon. Plants have used the light process of nature, outside the human being, to bind this element before we take it in with our food. Carbon, or coal (Rudolf Steiner referred to it as a dark, plebeian churl) must also pass the zero point of spiritualization. In the process it reveals something of its archetypal spiritual form, its light–like diamond aspect. This dark substance also holds within it the great cosmic Imaginations, creative cosmic images, and in the process of spiritualization, in becoming inner light, it stimulates the creative processes of the organism. It then condenses to human substance until it is finally exhaled. A resurrection process is thus active within us through carbon, though we are not consciously aware of this. It arises as a light that fashions organs, and this is closely connected with the process in which conscious activity of soul and spirit generates living, youthful light.

What happens to the light processes when cancer, the disease of our age that threatens us all, develops? Dr Clara Zupic, a pioneer of anthroposophical medicine in Yugoslavia who died a few years ago, wrote an important book, *Der Krebs als Lichtstoff-wechselstorung* (Cancer as a disorder of light metabolism). This was the fruit of a long life in medical practice and it contains important germinal thoughts. Let me present just the symptoms that are best suited to show the way in which cancer may be seen as a disorder of inner light processes, and also of warmth processes.

Four symptom complexes are particularly striking in the pre-cancerous states which generally persist for years:

1. A certain heaviness which may take the form of obesity, immobility, lack of elasticity, and also constipation and glandular and hormonal imbalance. The impression is that the organism is not fully breathed through and therefore also deficient in inner light.

2. Absence of febrile temperatures over many years; very low base temperatures and no proper relationship to one's own body temperatures, so that cold hands or feet are not even noticed.

3. Sleep disorders – the typical broken sleep. 'Asleep, human beings live in the light.' Having been awake and in their bodies for a long time, they long again for the lightness (or buoyancy) of light. The liberation felt on leaving behind the heaviness of the body, giving oneself up to the regenerative powers of the hier-archies, to the light, is constantly inter-rupted in pre-cancerous subjects; the spirit soul does not properly free itself, it falls back into the bodily state, as it were, and this means troubled sleep, with the individual waking up unrefreshed in the morning.

4. Finally, one commonly notes non-specific pain, now here, now there, sometimes concentrating on a particular organ,

though there appears to be nothing physically wrong. Here the astral body is not intervening the way it should; it gets stuck, jammed, and this should attract the physician's attention. If it is overlooked, a carcinoma will finally develop.

Psychologically the process of darkness is evident from a subtly depressive mood, which is not a clinical depression. This goes hand in hand with a certain lack of interest in the world around; the life of the senses is lukewarm, subdued. These patients often show a tendency to fold in upon themselves, reacting to anything new with anxiety. Added to this is the frequent inability to give expression to problems that weigh heavily on the mind and get rid of them by doing so. So the dark is swallowed down instead of being resolved through insight, in the light of awareness, and thus overcome. There are of course others who show a certain non-chalance, and may indeed appear quite offhand. Behind this, however, darkness is lurking; it is merely covered up with outward brightness.

When it comes to the spirit, we note that initiative lacks elan, and there is hesitation in the gesture of coming upright again after suffering an injury to the soul. Dr Schoch, an anthroposophical physician who died many years ago, presented an unforgettable picture on one occasion when he spoke of the 'hairy look' in a cancer patient's eye. The eyes express the intensity of our egoity, our inner light. In these patients they have lost their radiance. It is as if they yielded before the eyes of another person. The heavenly light of the spirit has become veiled.

Now the strange thing is that the darkness of the pre-cancerous state will often be seen to lighten when a tumour develops. This holds a certain danger, for it may prevent the early diagnosis of a cancer process which has now taken physical form. A kind of liberation occurs from the dark, intangible something, seeking here and seeking there, to which the patient has been subject for such a long time. The process has finally become localized. A valve has been created through which the proliferative energies can let off steam. Patients who brighten up like this when the tumour makes its appearance have a better prognosis than those who literally continue to have fear 'in their bones'; these will soon develop recurrences, with the dark heaviness never lifting.

The final act, the advanced tumour process, may come to expression in various ways. We all know the imploring eyes that say, 'Please, doctor, offer some hope!' The patient appeals to the inner light of the physician, being unable to produce his own. We also meet resignation and on the other hand rebellion, and these may alternate. Finally we may experience the final and most important element, that of saying yes to destiny, and a new inner light arising. This may be the fruit of the physician and the patient walking the same path together.

What is our therapeutic task when we face cancer, that most severe disorder of light metabolism? Let me give you just a brief outline, for these recommendations also point to ways in which mankind may overcome the disease for the future.

Mistletoe is *the* therapeutic agent in this case, for growing beyond the sphere of the dark forces of anti-Michaelic, ahrimanic spirits, it overcomes those powers in the course of its development. It interiorizes light and warmth to a much higher degree than other plants. So we may visualize these imponderables as a warm, golden stream that takes hold of the lightless, suffocative metabolism of the tumour and transforms it. The process is supported by all light-related substances such as phosphorus, magnesium, silica and iron, to mention just a few. At the same time it is important to stimulate warmth metabolism in every possible way, through warmer bedcovers and clothing, with the aid of baths and through remedial eurythmy.

For soul forces that have fallen into darkness, coloured light therapy, the life work of Dr N. Glas, the British physician who died recently, is an invaluable aid. As a young man he studied under Rudolf Steiner and was closely connected with him. The coloured light therapy he introduced appeals to conscious awareness, to the ego, and stimulates the essential qualities of sensory function – the sense of sight, of hearing, of touch, the sense of movement and of language. The after-images appearing in the complementary colours signify an objective process, filling the organism with form-creative powers. Coloured light therapy appeals to the etheric body, the bearer of all inner light. The colours are the deeds and sufferings of light in its struggle against darkness. Perception of colour also appeals to the astral body, however. When we see colour, we are connected with astrality. Colour therapy of any kind was referred to as therapy for the future by Rudolf Steiner.

Bringing light into the life of the soul also calls for all other forms of art therapy.

The guiding principle should be the setting of limits to, and hence a deepening of, sensory impressions.

Finally we must endeavour to let 'the reality within which we live,' as Dr Zeylmans came to call it from personal experience, come alive for our patients. This reality is not the world that presents itself to the senses, of course, but the presence, in the spirit, of the Christ, who has entered into the earth. When we experience Christ in the power to come upright again after suffering great pain, in the inner certainty, the inner equilibrium which comes when we obey the voice of conscience, in the sunlike clarity of thought which is the gift of the gods, we stand in light of the Christ power. As we gain insight in awareness into the way that Christ works within us, light will enter more and more profoundly into human nature, filling it with love and the sacred flame of enthusiasm. Slowly, very slowly, this will lead to the realization of an ideal for the future that Rudolf Steiner spoke of. Then carbon will not merely be eliminated as a gas but transformed in the inner light process, so that – like plants in a way – we shall no longer use oxygen but carbon dioxide, and use it to build up our bodies as we breathe. Then carbon will come close to its archetypal form in us, to being a transparent, light-filled diamond. That is the alchemical secret of the philosopher's stone which was uniquely brought to realization by Christian Rosenkreutz in the 13th century when his body became transformed and transparent and he experienced the event at Damascus and beheld the Risen Christ in a new way. This gave him the power to radiate the whole wisdom of the world that lives in light, in word and deed. The Christian Rosenkreutz impulse is still alive and active today and can be the ideal of all healing activity for us. In the beginning, God created the outer light. It is our task to create the living inner light. All the hierarchies are waiting for this. It is our responsibility to transform the earth through inner activity into the luminous star of our future existence.

CHAPTER 5

GIFTS OF EARTH AND COSMOS:
THE HEALING POWER OF ANTIMONY

Rudolf Steiner made certain statements relating to antimony that have encouraged
quite a number of anthroposophical doctors
and scientists to publish significant material
on the subject. The potential uses of
antimony as a medicinal principle are many,
however, and the mysteries of this metal are
far from fully explored. This paper presents
a further attempt to consider the essential
nature of antimony against the background of
the work that has already been done.

You may have the opportunity one day to
contemplate some crystals of stibnite (antimony glance), which is the most characteristic antimony ore. Observe the silvery rays
very carefully, enter into them, as it were,
and identify with them, and you may well
experience the tremendous dynamic of those
radiating crystals, a dynamic that takes you
all the way to the periphery. Yet you will
not be floating away on the air, the way
you might do when immersing yourself in the
scent of a lily; instead, you feel yourself
grow in inner strength, wholly awake, wholly
concentrated, feeling as if you were full of
the structural firmness that comes with
strength of purpose, even where your physical body is concerned. Anyone who has seen
one of the most magnificent specimens of
stibnite ever found, a mass of crystals
coming from Japan, with rays that are a
metre long and the thickness of an arm, may

recall the feeling of being almost shattered at first by the sheer power of this crystal-line form, and how that feeling then gave way to one of inner strength and clarity.

When we really want to get to know someone we try and find out their interests, the things they relate to and those they tend to avoid. We can use the same approach to find out about the nature of antimony.

The metal forms many compounds, particularly with sulphur. Stibnite, for example, is a sulphide of antimony. Sulphur also unites antimony with other metals, for instance with silver in pyrargite or red silver ore. Antimony forms compounds with all the halogens (fluorine, chlorine, bromine and iodine) and its great affinity to oxygen is evident from the fact that it forms many oxides. The colours of antimony ores and compounds range from yellow through all the reds to violet, and we can perceive the fiery side of this element in the rich play of colours and in the way it forms relationships with such ease. When we come to consider the wide variety of antimony compounds, some occurring naturally and some produced synthetically, we cannot but become freely mobile also within ourselves, taking great pleasure in the wide interests shown by this substance. It is not much given to forming salts, however, and chemically behaves either like a base or an acid, producing antimonates if reacted with bases and relatively unstable antimony salts with acids; overall there is a marked tendency to form complex salts.

The pure metal, elementary antimony, is a silvery white lustrous substance that is only rarely found in nature. It can be obtained by liquation, a process in which stibnite flows away from accompanying impurities. It is heated with scrap iron and a certain amount of potash and glauber salt until the antimony melts and can be run off from below the slag. The metal obtained by this method is often called antimony regulus, the antimony king. A star-shaped relief marks the surface to indicate its purity, and for this reason it is sometimes also called 'starry antimony king'. It forms silvery hexagonal rhombohedral crystals, like hoarfrost. The symbol used by alchemists for antimony regulus showed the earth surmounted by a crown:

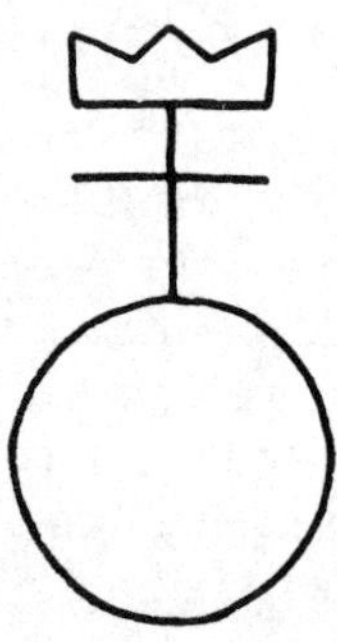

The star is of course merely an outward sign of the wholly crystalline, fern-like structure of this pure antimony. Plant-like forms like these are also produced when thin layers of antimony vapour are precipitated on to smooth surfaces under vacuum. If antimony combines with oxygen, of its own accord or on combustion, the resulting antimony trioxide shows flower- or snowflake-like forms. Pure antimony and its oxides thus do not show the spearlike conformation of stibnite, but a lively, rich and varied world of crystalline forms.

These observations have brought us closer to the essential nature of antimony as it comes to expression in form and gesture: the dynamic, spear-like radiance of stibnite; many different combinations formed with metals, halogens and oxygen; the crystalline structure of pure antimony, the starry king.

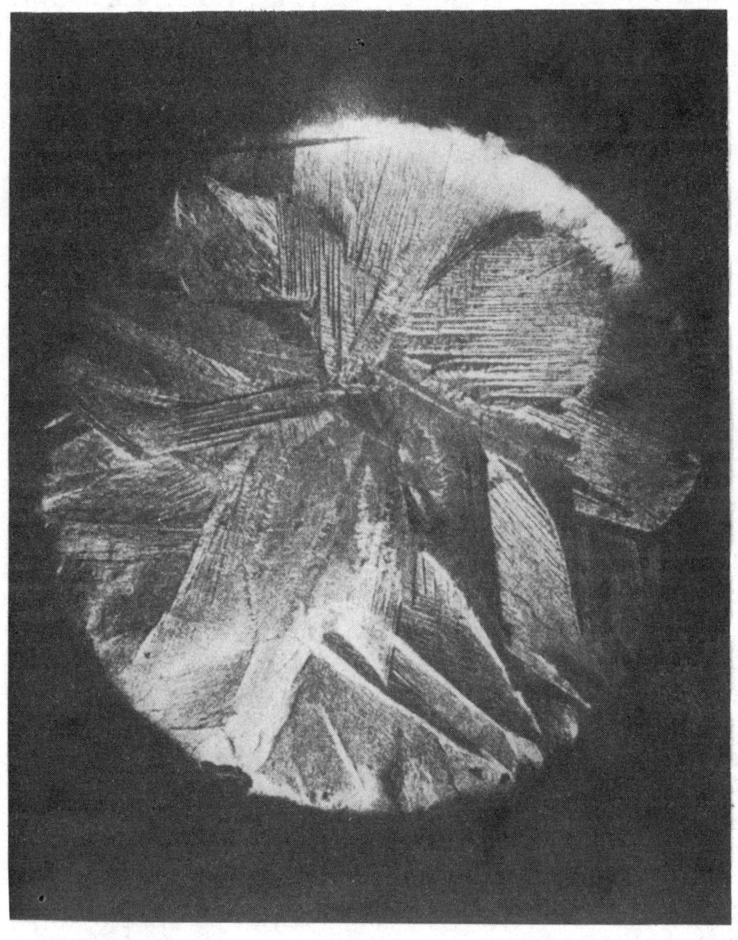

Cloos drew attention to the fact that antimony is most frequently found wherever a break occurs in the earth's crust and parallel displacement has led to tear faults. Such areas are found mainly in the Andes and Cordilleras, the rift valleys of East Africa, in southern Europe, including the Burgenland part of Austria, in Turkey, Southern Siberia, and above all in China and Japan. South Africa, China, Bolivia and Russia are the main antimony producers today. The metal is used to harden alloys for machine parts that are subject to great mechanical strain, axles and shafts for instance, and for the type of metal used by printers (antimony alloys expand as they solidify and are suitable for producing sharp casts of impressions). The metal is thus on the one hand swallowed up by machines, and on the other serves to feed the intellect. It is also used to remove traces of less precious metals in the purification of gold, binding them through sulphur. In the middle sphere, where healing has its place, present-day medicinal use is limited to anthroposophical medicine where it holds great promise for the future.

In the past it was a different story. During the Bronze Age, antimony was combined with copper, tin and lead in alloys used to make sacred vessels. The Persians fully appreciated its cosmic significance and celebrated the Feast of Antimony, with the metal playing a special role in the ritual. Sacred vessels made of pure antimony have been found that were made by the Chaldeans in the third millenium before Christ. Later, in Egyptian times, more worldly uses were found, and stibnite was used for make-up. The mineral came to be extremely popular in the Orient; it was ground to a black powder and made into kohl, an expensive cosmetic used for eye make-up. It emphasized the lustre of the eyes, their radiance and power of vision, and was considered an excellent protection against the 'evil eye'. The black paint could also be applied to achieve demonic effects, and the Prophet Ezekiel and later Tertullian, the early Christian writer, warned against the use of the 'devilish stuff'. The Persian poet Firdusi, who lived in the 10th century, wrote:

With paint to deepen dark eyes' shade,
Their glitter is demonic made.

When we consider the powerful radiance and centrifugal dynamics of stibnite, we can also see how an excess of this power may hold great dangers.

Medicinal uses of antimony go back a long way. It was used in ancient Egypt because of its drying properties and served to treat the eye inflammations that are so common in those regions, as a major styptic (to stop bleeding), and finally to prevent further tissue breakdown in running sores. The Egyptians called the metal *stem*, the Greeks made this into *stimmi*, and the Romans finally into *stibium*. Using it to treat eye conditions, the Greeks called it *plathyoph-thalmon*, 'eye widener', but the most beautiful name they had for it was *anthemonion*, 'come into flower'. Galen, the Greek physician of the 2nd century AD, used antimony to treat inflammations of the upper respiratory tract and the vagina. Later physicians, particularly the Arabs who practised in southern Europe, esteemed it most of all as a styptic in the treatment of nosebleeds and bleeding haemorrhoids, and for its cleansing, drying effect on proud flesh, polyps and rodent cancers.

Centuries followed when awareness of the medicinal powers of antimony were lost in a state of 'pralaya', until Paracelsus (1493-1541) brought it back into use in the 16th century, now going beyond purely external use and prescribing it also internally in a wide variety of different preparations. He sometimes combined antimony with plant extracts, and the mobile element in its many different variations willingly entered into such combinations. This was the beginning of chemistry, or iatrochemistry (medical chemistry), a tremendous and most courageous step to take at a time when the age of the Spiritual Soul was just beginning. It meant that Paracelsus was under serious attack from the University of Paris, a stronghold of the Arabian school, extremely conservative and bitterly opposed to the 'new chemical drugs'. Paracelsus did not waver, however. His '*mineralium, quorum summum, ac potissimum arcanum in se claudit Antimonium,* ' as he put it, – antimony holding the highest and most powerful of mysteries – was processed, using skilled spagyric methods, until the poison yielded medicaments which he prescribed very specifically on a number of indications. He thus initiated the rediscovery of the powers of antimony, though this was at a time when it could not yet be understood.

The result was that indiscriminate use led to many cases of poisoning and also death, and finally the notorious 'antimony dispute'. The University of Paris banned the use of antimony in 1566 and, from 1580 onwards, every candidate for a doctor's degree at Heidelberg University had to swear an oath that he would never prescribe antimony. In spite of this. famous physicians would run the risk of being struck off and continued to prescribe a great variety of antimony preparations because these had such comprehensive healing powers. Antimony was used to treat skin conditions, leprosy, the plague, asthma, pneumonia, malaria, stomach complaints and cancer, and also melancholia and epilepsy. Chartier said in 1640 that antimony was the most dangerous and at the same time the most effective drug. He called it the most magnificent remedy in the world, not only for humans but also for metals, for it removes all non-precious impurities from gold, acting as a 'philosopher's magnet' in drawing them out, or as a *'lupus metallorum'*, a ravenous wolf, in swallowing them up. It was therefore also called 'fiery dragon', 'the highest judge', or 'bath of kings'. Nevertheless, its use gradually declined again, though in 1838 Professor Sachs in Königsberg was to write: 'Antimony is indisputably one of the most effective and indispensable remedies, having a vitalizing effect on the stomach and intestines, the bronchial mucosa and the whole skin.' Antimony potassium tartrate (potassium antimonyltartrate containing variable amounts of tartar), or tartar emetic, was used in aversion therapy for mental conditions, and an ointment made with it, Ungt. Tartari Stibiati, served as a derivative, producing eruptions or pustules and drawing the disease process out into the skin. This ointment was also applied to the heads of the mentally ill.

At the beginning of this century, organic antimony compounds such as stibophen (fuadin) and sodium stibogluconate were produced and successfully used to treat tropical diseases: bilharziosis, filiariasis, kala-azar, leprosy, and also syphilis, worms, and foot and mouth disease. Being very toxic, they went out of use again, however.

Then came Rudolf Steiner. After centuries when knowledge of the powers of this substance had been in abeyance, he revealed the true nature of this most mysterious of all metals, giving it new life as a medicinal agent.

We began this chapter by trying to see what the gestures of antimony would tell us. Rudolf Steiner used spiritual science to gain insight on a higher level. In the first course of lectures he gave for members of the medical profession, antimony is mentioned in powerful terms:

> There are certain powers outside man that have an inner relationship to powers of the human will, and this is due to the fact that in the course of evolution in the kingdom of nature, the very last principle to be eliminated was the one that has to do with the conscious will. This was separated out last in the kingdom of nature.

Cloos confirms that the large antimony deposits did not form until the end of the Tertiary period, i.e. the middle of the Atlantean epoch.

Rudolf Steiner also referred to the fact that stibnite tends to crystallize in clusters. It aligns itself on the powers of crystallization that ray towards the earth in straight lines, on the deed of spirits from exalted regions of the universe. Reaching outward centrifugally, it tears itself away from the earth forces in the process. Rudolf Steiner therefore defined its structure as dynamite made manifest, or crystallized will. He said that in stibnite we could see the powers of crystallization that came from beyond the earth with our own eyes, and he called it a downright betrayer of those powers. Schwenk said on one occasion that essential nature and physical appearance were one and the same in stibnite, and this is something we can indeed experience.

In Rudolf Steiner's eyes, the marked affinity that antimony has for other metals and substances, particularly sulphur, is a very important characteristic of this medicinal agent. Sulphur creates the bridge which enables antimony to act on the protein process. We shall return to this later. In the many other compounds, some of which have been mentioned earlier, antimony unfolds its mercurial qualities, its youthful vitality. The inner fire of its nature is revealed in pyrargyrite, also known as *lapis ignis* (fire stone). According to Basilius Valentinus, fire is its quintessence. In berthierite, the structuring power of antimony is enhanced by iron. Stibnite provides the basis for many chemical compounds. It can be obtained from the gangue by the Seiger smelting process. If the molten ore is allowed to cool slowly, with air excluded, it crystallizes into fine fibrous structures, again showing a dynamic tendency to struggle free from the earth forces.

Pure antimony is a child of heaven. It does not like to show itself in physical form in nature. It can however be obtained by the liquation process that has already been described, after which evaporation brings it close to its primal state. If the volatile substance is then transfixed to a cold

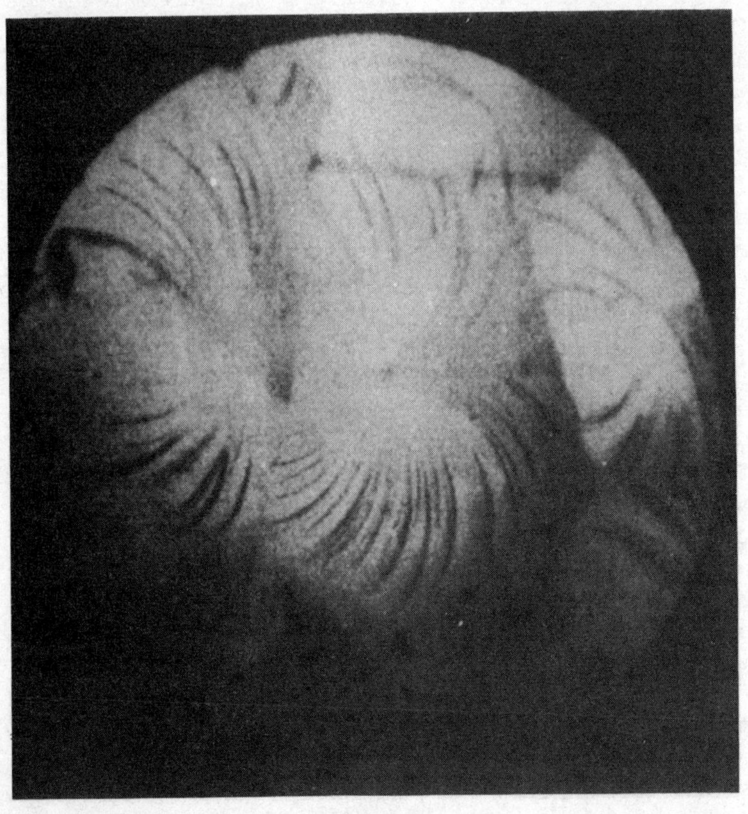

surface it will again reveal the cosmic
element in its crystalline nature. Rudolf
Steiner made repeated reference to the flowers
of antimony which form when the pure metal
is made red hot and the resulting white
antimony trioxide vapour precipitates on cold
surfaces. Particular importance however at-
tached for Rudolf Steiner to the mirror which
is formed when pure antimony is evaporated
under vacuum. Work done by Goetzberger
throws more light on the process. When a
mirror is produced by evaporating antimony
under vacuum, the metal first precipitates in

its amorphous form, forming very fine layers that are 180–250 angstrom in thickness (one angstrom equals the ten millionth part of a millimetre). As soon as the layer gets thicker, the gradual transformation of the amorphous metal into rhombohedral crystals starts from isolated centres of crystallization. The centres grow into discs at a constant rate and finally merge to form a new mirror, which sometimes shows a peculiar division into three. If more antimony is precipitated, and the thickness begins to exceed 2,000 angstrom, a totally different type of crystallization develops. It does so explosively, and individual crystals then no longer radiate from the centre but form concentric circles around it, again producing a mirror. The general impression is that, having been fettered in the amorphous form that had been produced by artificial manipulations, the metal uses all its strength to escape from the imposed non-crystalline form. The process is a slow one in thin layers but explosive in thick ones.

Antimony has one special property that Rudolf Steiner probably was the first to define; it rebuffs the sub-physical powers of electricity and magnetism. Antimony is diamagnetic, i.e. it places itself at right angles to the needle in a magnetic field and is pushed out of the field. The antipathy to electricity emerges when antimony compounds are subjected to eletrolysis. The metal is deposited on the cathode in its amorphous state, but as soon as it is touched with a pointed object there is a small explosion as the metal escapes from any coercion imposed by electricity.

Pure antimony in the form of the 'starry

king', in the form of flowers of antimony and, above all, in the form of the crystalline mirror has overcome the earth forces with their sub-physical components of electricity and magnetism, and enters into a living variety of form. The force of will shown by stibnite in its dynamic radiation here gives way to a tendency to produce rich variety of form, and this shows that there is a side to antimony that relates to thought activity. The Stibium met. praep. used in anthroposophical medicine comes from relatively thick mirrors that are entirely crystalline.

Rudolf Steiner thus provided the spiritual basis for present-day antimony therapy. He also said: 'The human being is antimony . . he actually is antimony.' Antimony is therefore intimately bound up with the processes that give rise to the human being.

We have noted that one and the same process produces antimony in nature and conscious will in human beings. This conscious will is an ego function, and we are thus able to understand the following words of Rudolf Steiner: 'Antimony processes introduced into the human organism act in the same way as the ego organization.' On the other hand antimony supports everything which – under the influence of unconscious powers of thought – has organizing functions in human beings, and that means the etheric body, which in the child is fully engaged in modelling, form-giving activities, and partly metamorphoses later to provide the basis for thought activity. Rudolf Steiner said: 'Antimony is very receptive to etheric powers. It nestles close to the etheric powers . . . With antimony we introduce something into the human organism that meets the activities of the etheric body half way.'

The above-mentioned paper by Goetzberger refers to an interesting fact. The configuration in which antimony crystallizes immediately brings to mind a drawing by Rudolf Steiner in his *Occult Physiology*. He was describing the etheric currents that arise when a memory image is formed in the brain. Like two electric currents of very high voltage that are in opposition, the etheric currents moving in the direction of the pineal gland are opposed to those arising from metabolism and moving towards the pituitary gland. When equilibrium is achieved between the two currents, a mental image has become memory and been imprinted on the etheric body. Antimony, a substance with affinity for the etheric, thus manifests in physical forms that reflect an etheric process.

Finally Rudolf Steiner said the following:

Powers similar to those of antimony have to be recognized in the astral body, and these act centrifugally, from the inside to the outside, in that organism . . . If antimony is introduced into the organism, the astral powers that are lacking are artificially produced.

This immediately brings stibnite to mind. On the other hand, antimony also helps the astral body to relate properly to the etheric body; it establishes a rhythmical relationship between these two bodies.

It will now be easier for us to understand Rudolf Steiner's statement that man, the way he is formed, really is antimony. This substance relates to the etheric and astral bodies and to the ego and it imposes form in the physical body. When a mediaeval alchemist made a homunculus, he projected his own albuminizing powers into the configuration of powers of evaporating antimony, creating a phantom of himself in a process that also helped him to gain self awareness.

Rudolf Steiner's description of the polarity between antimony and the albuminizing powers gives some indication as to the medicinal uses of this substance.

The processes in which albumin and other proteins are formed must be envisaged as swelling, burgeoning processes. They create form and dissolve it again and are the vitalizing and chemically active aspect of the life and sound ethers. If they were the only powers at work, however, we would end up as wobbly jellyfish. A structuring element must come in, so that individual organs can form, and this must have a relationship to the etheric if it is to be effective. Antimonizing powers are constantly at work in the organism, as artists modelling organ-forming substance to give it definite form. Light and warmth forces of the etheric world are active within them.

We can observe this in the blood. Blood is a substance that has a swelling life of its own, constantly coagulating to form organs, and on the other hand needing to be prevented from coagulating too much. Here we see the cooperation and mutual interaction between the natural antimonizing and albuminizing powers. Antimony represents a living interplay of powers that also exists in the healthy human organism. Haemophilia and other forms of bleeding from organs call for antimony, to prevent organs from melting and flowing away. 'These very antimony powers are active in the coagulation of the blood.

An anatomizing principle is at work there'
(Steiner). The coagulating principle is part
of the ego-related side of antimony, the ego
being a power that constantly works to
establish equilibrium. Antimony supports it
in its protein-forming and shaping activity,
a tendency that applies even at cellular
level. The albuminizing powers produce the
cell substance, they round out the cells,
whilst the centrosomes, which are produced
in the ovum after fertilization, use their
antimonizing power to bring order into the
process of cell division. This also explains
why antimony is important in cancer therapy,
when anti-antimonizing, structure-destroying
powers have gained the upper hand and led
to the undifferentiated proliferation of cells.

Diseases like typhoid, in the widest sense,
are another indication for antimony therapy.
Here one is dealing with an excess of foreign
protein that the ego and astral body have
not been able to cope with. The result is
ulceration and diarrhoea on the one hand,
fever and drowsiness on the other. Antimony
will strip the protein of its individual
powers, reducing it to a 'sensitive chaos',
as it were, so that it becomes amenable to
the structuring, function-inducing powers of
the ego organization and the astral body. A
'nerve-forming process in the wrong place'.
as Rudolf Steiner characterized typhoid fever,
is overcome when antimony restores the
constituent principles, which in this case are
going apart in a way that is appropriate
only to nerve development, to their proper
places. Antimony will therefore also cure
other ulcers in the digestive tract, it will
deal with inflammatory destruction in the
respiratory passages, and altogether be
suitable for the treatment of organs that are
growing friable.

External applications are used to treat eczematous and ulcerative skin conditions. Used in the form of ointments etc., antimony opposes the centrifugal action of certain powers in the astral body. Rudolf Steiner said that in this case the action of antimony was equivalent to that of sunlight at high altitudes, but that the same effect could also be achieved by pricking the skin with fine needles. It was important, however, to leave the antimony ointment or paste in place for as long as possible, under an occlusion dressing, until the organism took care of further development.

With regard to the potential side effects of antimony it has been said that this metal and its compounds have always been considered dangerous. Like the conscious will of man, it is dynamite made manifest. Excessively high doses given internally can cause patients to be overcome by an excess of formative powers, so that their organs have no strength left to carry out their functions in the digestion of food. Toxic doses cause vomiting and diarrhoea, malaise, collapse and even sudden death. Post-mortem examination will show vascular paralysis in the region of the splanchnic nerve, with corresponding cerebral anaemia. Rudolf Steiner recommended coffee as an antidote because it restored the proper rhythm between the organ-moulding powers and the organic processes in which food is assimilated. Caffeine does indeed dilate the vessels in the cerebrum, stimulate the respiratory and vasomotor centres, and cause the vessels in the splanchnic region to contract.

Rudolf Steiner prescribed a number of antimony preparations. Tartar emetic is the only one that he took from the past. Daems has written an excellent monograph on antimony in which he states that the preparation of tartar emetic goes back to the seventeenth century Rosicrucian pharmacist Adrian von Mynsicht who appears to be identical with the author of *Die geheimnen Figuren der Rosenkreuzer* (secret characters used by the Rosicrucians). He prepared it from tartar (Crocus metallorum – two parts of stibnite to one of saltpetre), a compound going back to Paracelsus, and caraway water, heating the whole in a sand bath. In small doses it acts as an expectorant and in larger doses as an emetic.

An important new medicine developed by Rudolf Steiner is Kalium aceticum cum stibio, which also contains saffron and red coral. It has proved highly effective in the treatment of conditions affecting the veins.

Stibnite/Anise ointment is prepared by an interesting method that was suggested by Rudolf Steiner. Antimonite is ground together with anise seed on a plate that is placed above a magnet. It is applied externally, with Cichorium in low potency taken internally afterwards, to treat certain gastric complaints.

Stibium metallicum praeparatum, the mirror preparation, is the one Rudolf Steiner prescribed most frequently. To prepare it, the metal is taken back to its original vaporous state in a process using fire, under exclusion of the earth-making oxygen. This may be regarded as a rebirth of the metal that is effected deliberately and with reverence, restoring it to a form that belongs to an earlier earth epoch when metals lived in a flowing variety of colour. When we use antimony in mirror form we may visualize it as a concentrate of cosmic powers that will activate all the constitutent principles and establish harmony among them.

The question finally arises as to the true nature of the antimonizing power. Rudolf Steiner described it as neutralized concerted action, a triad of Moon, Mercury and Venus powers. We may thus visualize the antimony sphere as extending from the earth to the sun. It encompasses the silver, mercury and copper spheres as it lovingly envelops the earth. The Risen Christ as painted by Grünewald in his Isenheim Altarpiece may be taken as an image of this sphere, a huge aura surrounding the head of Christ in Victory over Death, its gold, orange and red tones surrounded by a star-studded blue. This is the sphere that has given rise to antimony, a metal held by magic in the crystal spears of stibnite on earth. We begin to release it from its spell when we process it into a healing mirror, a metal that holds within it the power of resurrection.

Rebuffing the sub-physical powers it reveals itself as a metal of the future. We have to work with those sub-physical powers, but we will have to learn to manage them in such a way that they do not bind us in chains. We shall only be able to do this if we arm ourselves with 'super-nature', with the power of perceptive understanding that comes with spiritual training. The powers inherent in antimony can strengthen this.

Basilius Valentinus was clearly right in saying that antimony should be considered one of the seven wonders of the world and that there was no way in which a single individual could ever learn all about it, for life was too short. This chapter, too, must therefore inevitably remain fragmentary.

Looking once again at a stibnite crystal, or at the 'starry king', we see divine powers at work with our own eyes. Rudolf Steiner lifted the veil of mystery from this substance in such a way that his revelations are also a challenge to us to do further work, and continue in our exploration of the healing potential of antimony.

DR RITA LEROI

Born in Germany, the daughter of a journalist, Dr Rita Leroi attended the Stuttgart
Waldorf School and then went on to commer-
cial college. She worked as a journalist for
one year before taking up the study of
medicine. Following her marriage to Hans von
May, who was Swiss, she completed her
medical studies in Switzerland. Part of her
time as Clinical Assistant was spent at the
Ita Wegman Clinic in Arlesheim. During
eighteen years in general medical practice in
Basle she developed a profound interest in
the treatment of cancer and soon had the
care of many patients suffering from this
disease. In 1954 she married Dr Alexandre
Leroi, who was the Leader of the Society for
Cancer Research and Director of the Hiscia
Research Institute in Arlesheim, where the
mistletoe preparation Iscador is produced and
where research and development continue.

When the Lukas Klinik (St Luke's Clinic)
opened in Arlesheim in October 1963, Rita
Leroi became its director. On the death of
Alexandre Leroi in 1968 she also assumed the
directorship of the Hiscia Research Institute.
In 1978 Dr Leroi was elected President of the
International Anthroposophical Medical Associ-
ation, a position she held until her death on
8th September 1988.

In the course of the years she travelled
widely and gave many lectures on the
anthroposophical approach to cancer therapy,
where the whole human being is taken into
consideration, body, soul and spirit. This
aspect of her work took her to almost every

country in Europe, as well as to North and South America, India, New Zealand, Australia, Japan, South and South West Africa. Dr Leroi's published medical works and papers number about seventy.

WORKS BY RUDOLF STEINER FOR BACKGROUND
AND FURTHER READING:

Occult Science: an Outline , translated by G.
and M. Adams, Rudolf Steiner Press, London.

The Four Mystery Plays , translated Adam
Bittleston, Rudolf Steiner Press, London,
(particularly the play *The Guardian of the
Threshold*, reference to which is made in
Chapter 2).

Knowledge of the Higher Worlds , Rudolf
Steiner Press, London.

*The Bridge Between Universal Spirituality and
the Physical Constitution of Man* , translated
D. Osmond, (especially the lecture given on
18th December 1920) Anthroposophic Press,
New York.

An Occult Physiology , translation revised E.A.
Frommer, Rudolf Steiner Press, London.

Members of the medical profession may obtain
a list of medical titles by Rudolf Steiner and
other authors in German and/or English from:
The Society for Cancer Research, Kirschweg
9, CH 4144 Arlesheim, Switzerland.